The
Healing
Therapies
Bible

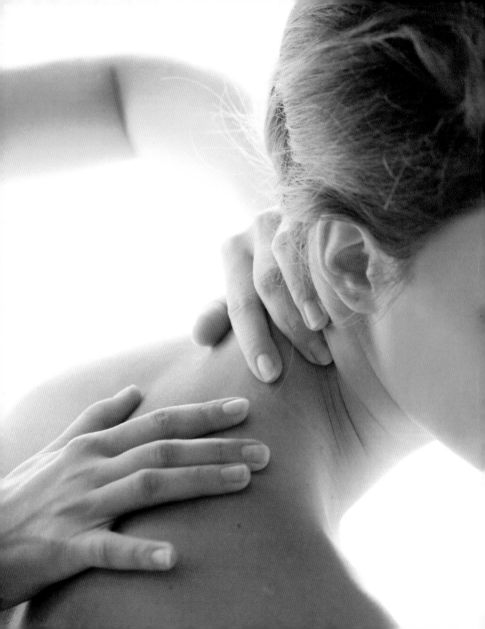

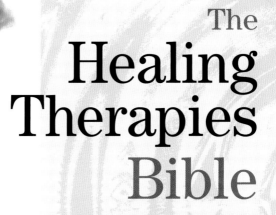

The
Healing
Therapies
Bible

Claire Gillman

Discover 70 therapies for
mind, body, and soul

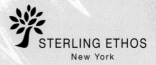

STERLING ETHOS
New York

Contents

Introduction   6

1 CLASSIC THERAPIES

Acupuncture   18
Massage therapy   24
Aromatherapy   30
Homeopathy   34
Osteopathy   38
Chiropractic   43
Hypnotherapy   47
Herbal medicine   53
Reiki   58
Reflexology   64
Nutritional therapy   69

2 MULTIDISCIPLINARY HEALING SYSTEMS

Ayurveda   74
Traditional Chinese Medicine   80
Naturopathy   85
Polarity therapy   90

3 POSTURAL/BODYWORK TECHNIQUES

Alexander Technique   96
Feldenkrais®   100
Dance movement therapy   105
Rolfing   109
Bowen therapy   113
Craniosacral therapy   116
Shiatsu   120
Qigong   125
T'ai chi ch'uan   129
Tui na Chinese massage   135

4 BREATHING TECHNIQUES

Rebirthing breathwork   142
Transformational Breath®   148
Buteyko   151
Holotropic Breathwork™   156
Holographic breathing   164

5 HEALING THROUGH THE SENSES

Art therapy   170
Colour therapy   173
Iridology   180
Bates method   185
Therapeutic sound therapy   191
Hydrotherapy   197

Light therapy 203
New-generation flower
    essences 210
Music therapy 216
Magnet therapy/electromagnetic-
    field therapy 220
Auricular therapy 225

6 ENERGY OR VIBRATIONAL HEALING

Kinesiology 232
Angelic reiki 238
Energy medicine 244
The BodyTalk System™ 250
Dowsing therapy 254
Zimbaté 258
Divine empowerment 262
Metatronic Healing® 266
Quantum-Touch 271
Chakra healing 276
The Journey 284
ThetaHealing® 288

7 PROGRESSION AND REGRESSION THERAPIES

Past-life regression therapy 296
Past-life integration therapy 300
Future-life progression 304
Akashic Record therapy 310

8 MIND AND PSYCHOLOGICAL TECHNIQUES

Sophrology 318
Meditation 322
Psychotherapy 328
Neuro-linguistic programming 335
Emotional freedom techniques/
    tapping 339
Picture-tapping technique 344
Matrix reimprinting 349
Compassion-focused therapy 353
F**k It therapy 358
Cognitive behaviour therapy 363
Cosmic ordering 368
Quantum-field healing 374
Biodynamic therapy 378

Useful contacts 384
Index 391
Acknowledgements /
    Picture credits 398

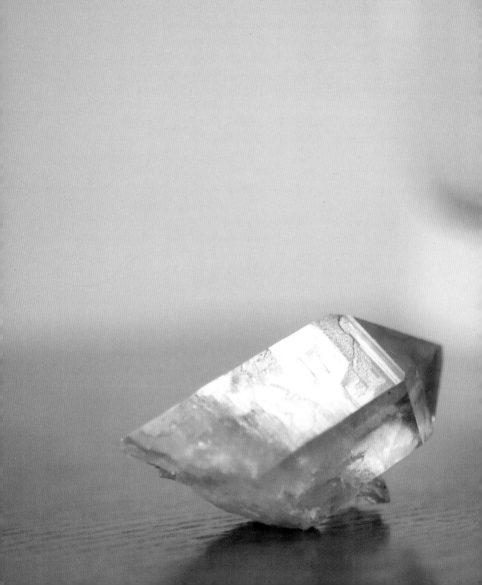

INTRODUCTION

Introduction

Healing therapies have brought relief from pain and improvements to the everyday lives of millions of people, young and old, all over the world. While many therapies offer relaxation, greater balance, or a chance to manage an illness or symptoms more effectively, some therapies have seen astonishing results in restoring people's health and well-being.

Most therapies treat body, mind, and spirit, and are devoted to bringing harmony to all three aspects of your life. There has never been a time when there have been so many healing therapies from which to choose, and fresh therapies are constantly emerging, while others are accelerating, using new-generation energies and techniques. More and more people are now becoming open to the wonderful possibilities of these healing modalities.

Healing therapies are no longer the preserve of the fringe minority. While 38 per cent of Americans and at least 25 per cent of people in England have used complementary or alternative therapy in the past year, that figure jumps to 52 per cent in Australia, and 85 per cent of Australians say they have used Complementary and Alternative Medicine (CAM) treatments during their lifetime.

More astonishing is the fact that, in one recent survey, 85 per cent of medical students, 76 per cent of physicians, and 69 per cent of hospital doctors said that they feel that complementary therapies should be made more widely available as part of general healthcare practice. This more integrated attitude to healing is benefiting those who seek a more holistic (whole-person) approach to health, and those who want to move away from some of the side-effects of allopathic medicine (mainstream Western medical

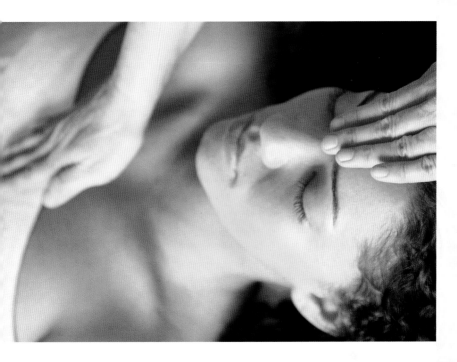

Energy therapists are now working with new higher chakras.

practice, which combats disease using drugs or surgery) and treatments. A more enlightened and integrated approach is gradually replacing the old scenario, in which conventional medicine was set against complementary therapies.

And this is an exciting time to be interested in alternative and healing therapies. There is a belief in the mind–body–spirit world that new healing modalities are arising to help us deal with, and ascend to, the higher planetary frequency that we are experiencing due to the "shift" of 2012 – an extraordinary spiritual awakening for humanity

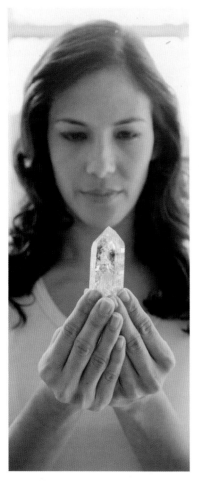

New higher-vibration crystals have appeared since the time of the spiritual "shift" of 2012 (see page 9).

and the planet, and a shift in consciousness (see also page 276). Along with this, therapies and remedies that took hold in the mid-1980s are now entering a new generation. Crystal healers have begun to work with new high-vibration crystals (see page 276), while flower-essence practitioners now have access to higher-vibration flower remedies (see page 210). And today a healing session may see a therapist working with the higher chakras (energy centres) – the chakras in the energy field – as well as with the seven chakras on the body (see page 176). These techniques are all becoming more widely available to us as we evolve spiritually.

Innovative techniques

New healing techniques are now being taught all over the world. Some are related to a particular healer, such as Brandon Bays's The Journey (see page 284), Vianna Stibal's ThetaHealing® (see page 288), and the BodyTalk System™ developed by Dr John Veltheim (see page 250). Others are generic and have evolved from a wealth of traditions – such as mindfulness meditation (see the box on page 326), with its roots in Buddhism and Western stress-reduction techniques; and regression therapy (see page 296), which was recently popularized by Harvard psychiatry professor Dr Brian Weiss.

This book profiles 70 different healing therapies, explaining the principles on which they are based and their history in practice, and, wherever possible, showing them in action. To kick off the book, we look at some of the classic techniques of complementary therapy, such as acupuncture, homeopathy, aromatherapy, and herbal medicine; and then at ancient multidisciplinary healing

Many people are experiencing a greater interest in healing therapies and a spiritual awakening.

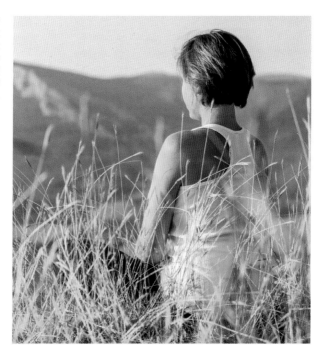

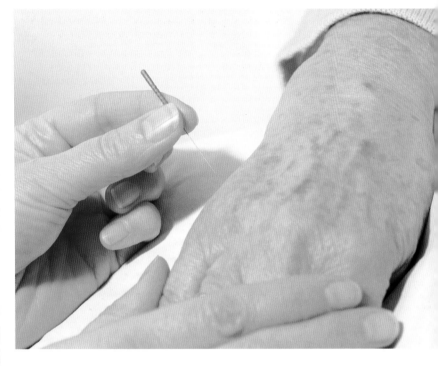

systems, such as Ayurveda and
Traditional Chinese Medicine
(TCM), with which you may
already be familiar. Subsequent
therapies are then divided into
chapters that loosely classify
them into:

- Postural/bodywork techniques
- Breathing techniques

*Traditional therapies such as acupuncture
are currently enjoying a renaissance.*

- Modalities that heal through
  the senses
- Energy or vibrational healing
- Progression and regression
  therapies
- Mind and psychological
  techniques.

How to use this book

If you are drawn to a particular genre of healing therapy, such as postural/bodywork techniques, then you will naturally want to dive into that chapter first. However, those of you who are simply interested in finding out what is available, and the developments that are occurring in various fields, will enjoy dipping in and out wherever a therapy catches your eye and seems to hold appeal. You do not need to read this book from cover to cover (unless that suits you), but can cherry-pick whatever therapy draws your attention, perhaps comparing it with similar therapies within that genre. Choosing a suitable healing therapy for yourself relies greatly on intuition and instinct.

The entries for each healing therapy are fairly comprehensive, but nothing beats trying it out for yourself, to see if it resonates well with you and whether you think it could be of help to you. You can start by looking at the websites of the many healing organizations and official bodies that are listed in the Useful Contacts section of this book (see page 384). It will give you a starting point from which you can then explore further.

Finding a therapist

Whichever healing therapy you choose to undertake, it is important that you find a suitably qualified practitioner.

One common concern, for those new to healing, is the difficulty of regulating such a varied range of treatments. However, most forms of healing and complementary therapy have one or more governing body which sets the standards for the training and services provided, as well as the codes of conduct for practitioners. Where the healing modality is pioneered by a particular healer and is not widespread, the best way to find a suitably qualified therapist is through the founder's website. The web addresses of governing bodies, as well as the luminaries of smaller healing modalities, can be found at the back of this book in the Useful Contacts section (see page 384).

Of course one of the very best ways to find a good practitioner is through word-of-mouth. However, in the absence of a recommendation – and even if you find a therapist through the professional governing organization – you should always check that the therapist is insured and request proof of their qualifications. It's also a good idea to ask about their experience

There are lots of new modalities to explore within the talking therapies.

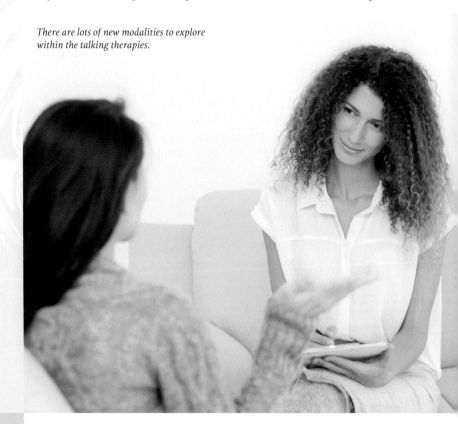

in treating people with similar conditions to your own.

Once you have established the therapist's credentials, the most important thing is that you feel comfortable with your chosen practitioner and have faith in their abilities. The healer–client relationship is a very important one, and from the outset you should feel relaxed and confident.

Medical advice

Healing therapies are highly effective at treating individuals in a holistic way, but they are not a substitute for medical advice. Many doctors now recognize the benefits of healing therapies, and you should discuss your intention to see a complementary therapist with your physician or health practitioner, and continue to take any prescribed medication. If you are pregnant, breast-feeding, or have any underlying health problems, you should inform your therapist before complementary treatment commences.

COSTS

Some healing therapies may be available as part of your country's health service, but for most of the modalities mentioned in this book you should expect to pay privately for treatment. It is worth enquiring about the cost of a healing session before booking, and you may wish to get a rough idea of how many sessions might be required (although this is, of course, always going to be a ballpark figure, depending on your own requirements and how you respond to treatment).

If you have private medical insurance, it is worth enquiring whether your policy covers your chosen therapy, because an increasing number of healing modalities are now eligible.

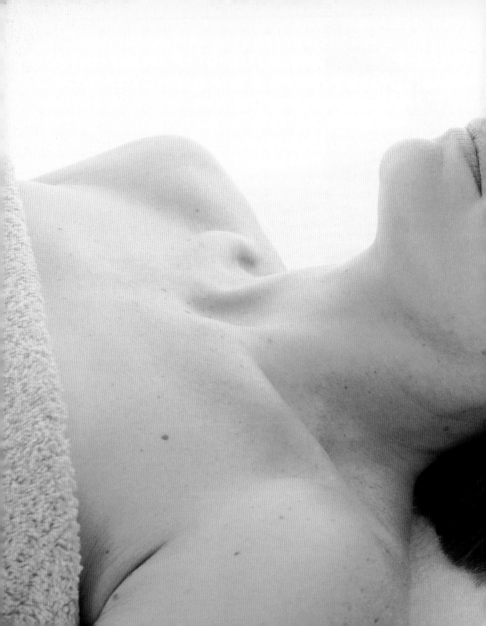

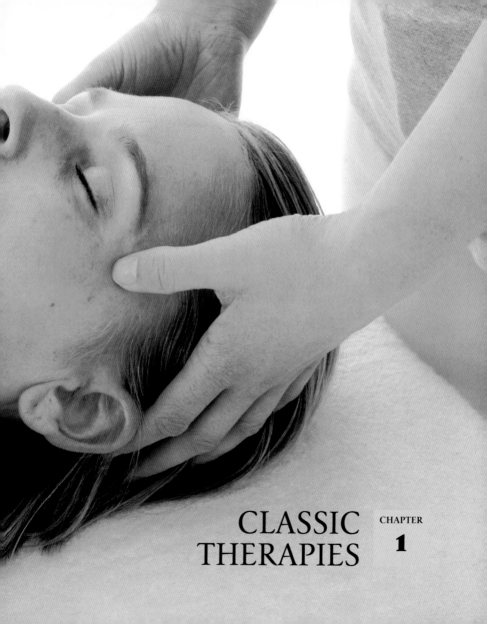

CLASSIC THERAPIES

CHAPTER 1

Acupuncture

Acupuncture is one of the modalities that is part of Traditional Chinese Medicine (TCM, see page 80) and other oriental medicines, but it has been popular in the West for at least 30 years.

Most people are familiar with the fact that it involves the insertion of fine needles into specific points on the body to stimulate the flow of energy (*qi*, pronounced "chi") along meridian lines (or energy

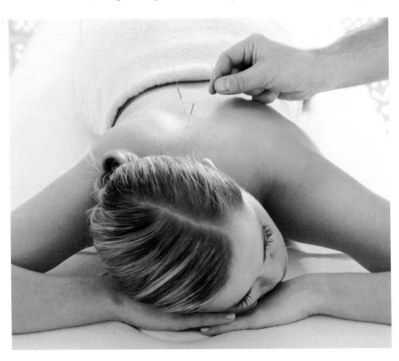

pathways) and to clear blockages. It is also known to release endorphins and enkephalins – the body's natural "feel-good" hormones – to ease pain and produce a "high".

History

It is believed that acupuncture originated from the observations by Chinese physicians of how various sword, spear, and knife wounds created different changes, depending on where on the warrior's body they were inflicted.

Who can benefit?

Acupuncture can be used for both physical and emotional difficulties, and is often sought out for dealing with addictions. It is especially effective for pain and stress relief, headaches, bowel, menstrual, and fertility problems, and difficult skin conditions. It is appropriate for all, including the old, the young (see the Acupressure box on page 21), and pregnant women. In fact many

Needles may be placed on areas of the body that are not affected by your condition.

pregnant women use acupuncture to help with morning sickness and to relieve back and sciatic pain, constipation, and heartburn; it is also used to help turn a baby who is presenting bottom-first (a breech birth) and to induce an overdue labour.

What to expect

You should turn up for your first appointment wearing loose clothes, so that the practitioner can insert the needles with ease. You will be asked for a medical history, and about your diet, sleep patterns, and emotional state. The practitioner will probably examine your tongue, check your skin colouring and type, take your pulses, and examine your body for posture, movement, and signs of muscle-tensing.

Once a treatment plan has been decided upon, you will be asked to lie on a massage table, and fine needles will be inserted at various points on your body and face to stimulate the *qi*. Don't be surprised if the places where the needles are inserted are not close to the site of your problems; for

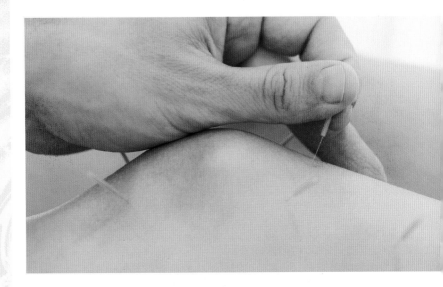

example, the acupuncture points to stimulate labour are found on the ankles and hands. There are 12 principal meridians that carry the body's energy, each corresponding to an organ or a function of the body. In addition there are two main meridians: the Conception vessel and the Governor vessel.

The number of needles to be inserted varies, depending on the individual case. They are left in place for a short time before being removed, and then you are allowed to relax and enjoy

In Japanese and Korean acupuncture, the depth to which the needles are inserted is generally shallower than in Chinese acupuncture. In all techniques, how deeply the needles are inserted depends on the area of the body and the condition being treated.

some peaceful contemplation, usually with dimmed lights and soft music. Occasionally the practitioner will apply movement to the needles. The process of inserting and removing them is painless, and you should not experience any discomfort throughout the treatment.

ACUPRESSURE FOR CHILDREN

Acupuncture is safe when used on babies and children, and some practitioners specialize in paediatric care. When treating children, the practitioner uses fewer needles (usually about four), leaving them in for a shorter period of time and being extremely gentle. However, many parents prefer to opt for acupressure when it comes to children (as do those with a fear of needles), because it is non-invasive.

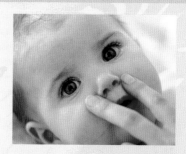

Acupressure is highly effective on babies and infants and massaging acupressure points can help babies get to sleep.

Acupressure is based on the same healing principles as acupuncture, but instead of inserting needles, the practitioner uses finger or thumb pressure only, to harmonize the energy flowing through the body (see also Shiatsu on page 120). The pressure can be gentle or firm, and is used to treat the same conditions as acupuncture; in addition, it can be used at home as a self-treatment, and as a great way to relieve pain such as headaches and backache, or cramps. If you want to use acupressure for self-help or to give it to members of your family, the acupressure points and massage are easy to learn and highly effective. The points and meridians correspond to those found on acupuncture charts, and they are pressed for at least 20 seconds, using the thumb, index, or middle finger. The degree of pressure varies, according to the condition, as does the direction in which you press: clockwise or anticlockwise.

MOXIBUSTION

Another practice in keeping with acupuncture (and sometimes used in conjunction with it) is the less well-known technique of moxibustion, which is also part of TCM. In moxibustion, a small quantity of a herb called moxa (or mugwort: *Artemisia vulgaris*) is applied to the end of an acupuncture needle while it is in place, and is then lit; or a small stick or cone is placed directly on the skin, and removed before the skin can burn. Moxibustion can be used as a treatment to help move stagnant *qi*, or in a diagnostic way to indicate where the body's energies need warming or "tonifying" (to strengthen the energy in a system).

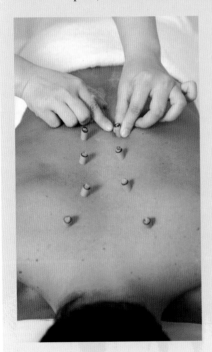

Moxa cones are made from the herb mugwort, which is excellent for pain relief.

SELF-HELP: if you are going to treat yourself or a friend with moxibustion, the most convenient form to use is a moxa stick, which you can buy from oriental medicine stores. It is easiest to light the stick from a candle (which can take some time), then hold the lit end about 2.5cm (1in) above the skin over the acupressure point. The sensation of warmth should be pleasant and relaxing. The stick should be temporarily removed and then returned (dabbing), if the sensation of heat becomes uncomfortable. There will be a strong smell of burning herbal smoke, which is not unpleasant, but can be overwhelming if the room is not ventilated.

A moxibustion session should last about 15–20 minutes. Be careful not to overheat the skin (which should only become slightly pink), and take great care when extinguishing the moxa stick – stubbing it out rarely works, as it tends to continue to smoulder; it is best to cut off the tip with a sharp knife on a board, when you have finished the session.

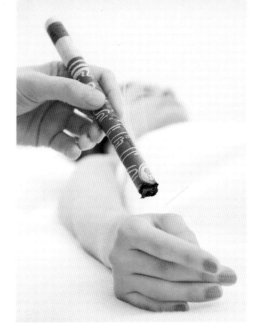

Hold the moxa stick about 2.5cm (1in) from the skin over the acupressure point.

CAUTION

The use of moxa is contraindicated (inadvisable for medical reasons) if you are pregnant, have high blood pressure, or broken skin; during acute illness (especially involving a raised temperature or inflammation); and on sensitive parts of the body such as the face.

Massage therapy

The relaxation and healing powers of massage have been well documented over the past 5,000 years. Extensively used in ancient Mediterranean civilizations to lessen pain and prevent illness, massage involves the manipulation of the soft tissues in the body, usually after applying oils, which may or may not be scented.

There are many different branches of massage, some of which are drawn from body therapies such as Rolfing (see page 109) and shiatsu (see page 120).

History

Despite its ancient origins, massage really came to wider popularity in the West after the introduction of Swedish massage in the 19th century by Per Henrik Ling (1776–1839), a Swedish fencing master. And the introduction of therapeutic massage, which took an overall holistic approach, kept massage in the popular eye during the 1970s as a way to promote overall good health.

STUDY FACT

In ancient Greece, anatripsis (the practice of rubbing up the limbs) was performed to treat fatigue as well as sports or war injuries.

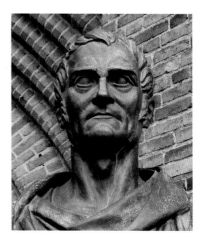

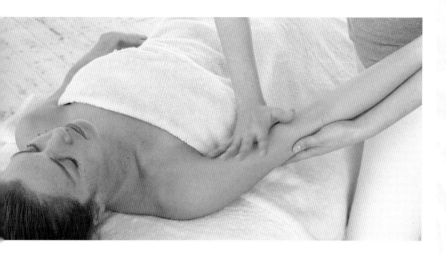

Above Massage for relaxation works through all the major muscle groups of the body.

Opposite Per Henrik Ling is the Swedish fencing master acclaimed for introducing the technique of Swedish massage.

Who can benefit?

Massage is generally used to induce relaxation, but it can be just as effective at working on the mind as it is on the body, and is highly beneficial in reducing the effects of stress, anxiety, or depression. It is also effective in treating people who suffer from high blood pressure, headaches, insomnia, and heart/circulatory problems. However, it is probably best known for treating neck and back pain, especially for those who spend long hours working at a computer keyboard.

What is less widely documented is the fact that massage can be used preventatively. A routine massage treatment is one of the best ways to prevent the onset of stress-related illnesses or injury from sport and exercise.

What to expect

A massage session usually takes place in a warm room, with the client lying on a massage table, although some practitioners favour working on the floor, often using a futon-style firm mattress. You will be asked to strip down to your underwear. A massage generally lasts 20–60 minutes.

The therapist will work with a base oil on their hands, to reduce friction and keep the massage movements smooth and flowing. Sometimes essential oils are added for their therapeutic effect (see Aromatherapy on page 30). The practitioner may use a range of strokes, which vary from gentle stroking (*effleurage*) and kneading (*petrissage*) to pressure (friction) and drumming (*tapotement* or percussion) – which itself ranges from drumming the fingers to vigorous chopping movements with the whole hand.

It is worth experimenting with different styles of massage, and different practitioners, until you find which particular massage strokes and essential oils suit you. Whichever style you favour, ultimately the experience should feel pleasant and relaxing, even if the massage is performed in an invigorating way.

The benefits of massage can be felt for hours or even days afterwards, and this treatment is especially beneficial when used in conjunction with other therapies.

MASSAGE WITH A PARTNER

This is a wonderful way to help release tired, aching muscles, while simultaneously being a sharing and giving part of your relationship. There are basic massage courses that you can attend as a couple or individually, and books and DVDs that you can follow. However, if you follow your instincts and let your hands stay as relaxed as possible, simply stroking, rubbing, and kneading each other gently can work fine. Above all, enjoy the massage and the intimacy.

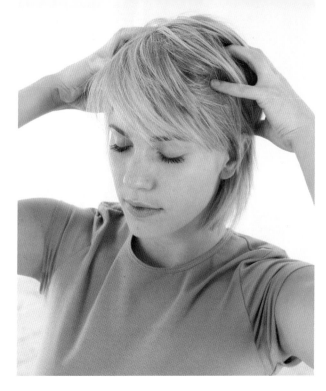

Self-massage techniques are easy to learn but even just rubbing wherever you feel tension in the body can help.

Self-massage

Massage on yourself can be highly effective and is easy to perform, when you have a spare moment. In fact many of us use self-massage unconsciously, whenever we rub a tense muscle or soothe our temples to ease a headache. Squeezing and kneading one shoulder after the other, massaging the palms of your hands and stretching your fingers, gently squeezing your neck muscles and the upper arms, and "working" the muscles of your thighs and calves are all good self-massage routines that will help to renew your energy levels and prevent the build-up of aches and pains.

MARMA MASSAGE

In Ayurveda (see page 74), the ancient system of Indian medicine, the fingers are used to massage the 107 marma points (vital points) throughout the body, to promote physical and mental healing and well-being.

A marma massage increases blood flow to the muscles surrounding each point, and can result in increased levels of energy, reduced stress, and freedom from tension and anxiety. Marma massage is good for relieving symptoms such as muscular pain and stress-related conditions, and is particularly beneficial to stroke victims.

During a session the marma therapist will check the acidic levels of your tongue with litmus paper (you are aiming for 60 per cent alkaline to 40 per cent acid, for optimum health), as well as checking your muscle and nerve reflexes. You can expect a course of between two and six weekly sessions, depending on your condition.

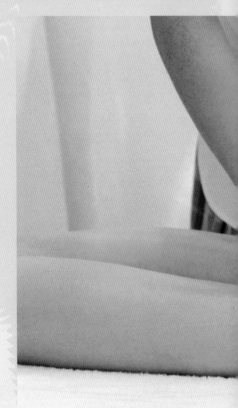

Marma massage focuses on 107 marma points (vital points) throughout the body.

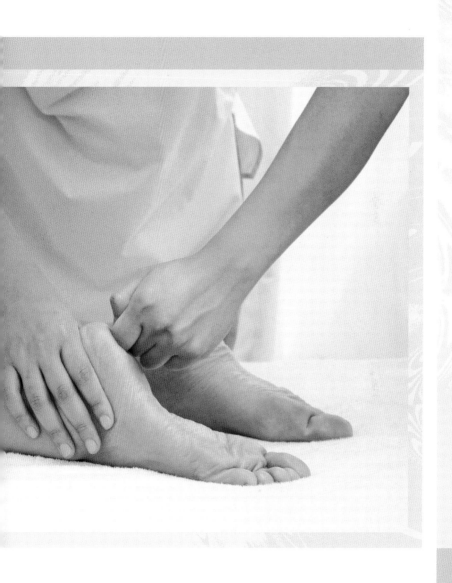

Aromatherapy

Aromatherapy uses highly concentrated plant oils (see the box below) to promote physical and psychological well-being. This method of healing has been in use since ancient times. Today, essential oils are used to treat a wide range of ailments and are well known for their effect on the emotions and mental well-being. And new-generation flower essences (see page 210) are being used to aid spiritual development, too.

Fragrance is the key element of aromatherapy, because smell has a direct effect on the brain and central nervous system, influencing our moods and feelings, relaxing the body and mind, and promoting self-healing. The oils can be used to fragrance a room by means of a vaporizer or oil burner: a reservoir is filled with water, to which you add a few drops of essential oil; the

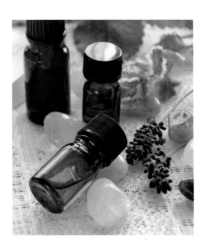

Essential oils are stored in dark coloured bottles as this filters out the sun's ultraviolet rays and preserves the effectiveness and longevity of the oils.

STUDY FACT

Essential oils are highly concentrated. It can take as many as 5,000 roses to produce just one teaspoon of essential oil.

reservoir is then heated and as the water heats up it evaporates, releasing the perfume of the warm oil. Another pleasant way to enjoy the effects of aromatic oils is to put one or two drops into a bath, just before you get in; the oil forms a thin film over the surface of the water, which coats and penetrates the skin as you lie there taking in the gorgeous aroma.

However, when essential oils are used directly on the skin (always diluted by a pure vegetable-base oil) in the form of massage, you get the additional benefit that they stimulate the acupuncture/acupressure points, the blood, and the lymphatic circulation, as well as calming the nervous system. In addition, oils applied directly to the skin are easily absorbed into the bloodstream and efficiently metabolized by the body.

History

There are writings from Egypt, China, and Persia – the oldest dating back at least 3,000 years – that document the ancient use of plant essences by priests, physicians, and healers. There are

WHAT ARE ESSENTIAL OILS?

Any part of a plant can be used to produce essential oils, and the method of extraction depends in each instance on the accessibility and site of the essence. Plant oils are produced in minute quantities by oil glands in the plant, and to harvest appreciable amounts, large quantities of plants need to be subjected to steam distillation (whereby the oil vaporizes into the steam), solvent extraction (where use of a centrifuge is followed by low-temperature distillation), or maceration (where the plant is soaked in hot oil and, as the plant cells collapse and release their essential oils, the mixture is separated and purified by a process called *defleurage*; if fat is used rather than oil, the process is called *enfleurage*).

CAUTION

Aromatherapy can be very effective, but the essential oils contain powerful active constituents, which may not mix well with other medical treatments. Ask your practitioner for advice, and always tell your aromatherapist about any medication or treatments that you may be having.

Similarly, certain aromatherapy oils are not recommended for pregnant women, so you should tell your therapist if you are pregnant, especially during the early months.

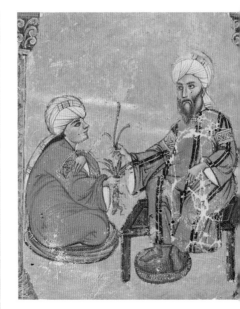

The oldest writings on plant essences date back at least 3,000 years.

also countless references in the Bible to the importance and high value that was attached to such essences.

Who can benefit?

Although best known for promoting relaxation and a sense of well-being, aromatherapy can also be used to treat illness. Each essential oil has a highly complex pharmacological structure, with a wide variety of uses. Some oils are anti-inflammatory and sedative; others stimulate the circulation or have anti-viral and immune-stimulating properties. Accordingly, aromatherapy has seen good results in treating:

• Wound-healing
• Skin conditions such as acne

- Menopausal and menstrual complaints
- Chronic fatigue
- Neck and back pain
- RSI (repetitive strain injury)
- Insomnia
- Anxiety
- Colds and flu
- Poor circulation
- Respiratory problems
- Stress and headaches.

Training

There are a number of recognized aromatherapy organizations worldwide, all of which should offer training and qualifications. If you want to sign up for training, make sure that your tutor and course are recognized by the governing body in your own country, which will oversee accreditation standards.

POPULAR ESSENTIAL OILS AND THEIR USES

NAME OF OIL	THERAPEUTIC USES
Eucalyptus	Colds, flu, rheumatism
Lavender	Acne, eczema, insect bites, minor wounds, insomnia, tiredness
Rose	Insomnia, pre-menstrual tension (PMT), scarring
Neroli	Frayed nerves and upset stomachs; good for dry skin
Tea tree, pine, lemon	Sore throats, colds, bronchitis; also a great antiseptic
Roman chamomile	Anxiety, stress, allergies, PMT
Geranium	Skin problems, neuralgia, tonsillitis
Patchouli	Dry skin patches and dandruff
Jasmine, melissa	Mood-enhancement

Homeopathy

This is a system of treatment (founded by the German doctor Samuel Hahnemann in 1796) which works on the principle that "like may cure like" – which is similar to the medical theory underlying vaccination or immunization. Homeopathy is said to stimulate the body's own healing processes to cure the particular ailment or overpower the bacteria, rather than treating the symptoms themselves. By introducing a remedy that mimics the symptoms, homeopathy builds up the body's resistance.

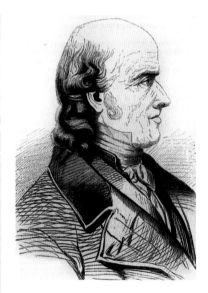

The German doctor Samuel Hahnemann founded the system of homeopathy in the late 18th century.

Homeopathy is widely practised in Europe, India, the US, and South Africa, often by conventionally trained physicians. In the UK, Queen Elizabeth II has (in addition to her two orthodox physicians) a specialist in homeopathy on her medical staff.

Homeopathic remedies use extracts from plants, minerals, salts, and animals. These extracts are dissolved and then diluted many times in alcohol or water (using a special technique) to form the remedies. Although you can buy homeopathic remedies over the counter, a homeopath will devise a remedy specifically for you, and it may contain a combination of substances.

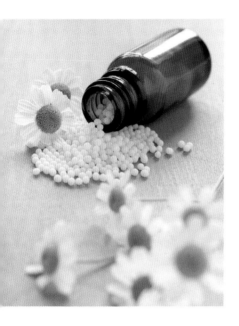

The active ingredients of homeopathic remedies are diluted (or "potentized") so that only a minute amount remains.

Such remedies should not cause any side-effects and you cannot become addicted to them. This is because only a very minute amount of the active ingredient is used, in a specially prepared form. Dilution of the remedy, accompanied by vigorous shaking, has a potentizing effect (that is, it makes the remedy stronger), and homeopaths believe that the more dilute the concentration, the more powerful and effective it is. This is one of the aspects of homeopathy that many orthodox doctors find hard to accept.

Who can benefit?

Homeopaths emphasize that they treat people, rather than diseases, and that a human being is more than the sum of his or her physical parts. Homeopathic medicine is said to be suitable for both acute and chronic conditions, and is safe even for young children

– a homeopath can prescribe remedies for babies suffering from problems such as colic, administering the medicine via a sweet pill, a powder, or a liquid.

Homeopathy can be used to treat a wide range of conditions and is especially effective for:

• Skin complaints
• Tiredness and chronic fatigue
• Allergies
• Hormonal problems, including the menopause
• Depression
• Breathing difficulties
• Stress and anxiety.

What to expect

In order to find the right remedy for you as an individual, your homeopath needs to know all about you. A detailed understanding of who you are – along with any illnesses, and details of how you experience them – is necessary to assess your case correctly. Finding out about your general energy levels, your past medical history, and the way you live is also important. This initial consultation may last an

hour or more. Your homeopath will then give you a homeopathic remedy, usually in tablet form, but occasionally as a powder or a liquid remedy. Subsequent appointments will last for about 30 minutes.

During the period of your treatment you may experience feelings of exceptional well-being and optimism. Conversely, you may get a cold, rash, or some form

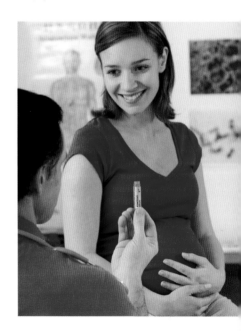

of discharge, which means that your system is going through a cleansing stage. Sometimes your symptoms can appear to get worse for a short time, but this is simply a sign that the remedy is taking effect. If any response to your treatment concerns you, contact your homeopath straight away. You may also want to make notes of any bodily or mental changes, and take them with you to discuss at your next appointment.

The length of homeopathic treatment depends on the individual. As a general rule, acute conditions respond more quickly, and the longer you have had a chronic illness, the longer it will take to disappear.

If you are given homeopathic remedies to take at a later date, be sure to store them in a cool, dark place, away from anything with a strong smell. If you travel, do not let your remedies go through the X-ray scanner at airports because it may degrade them.

At a time when conventional medicines are no longer an option, homeopathy is often chosen by pregnant women as an effective way to alleviate pregnancy ailments.

HOME FIRST-AID KITS

Many parents are now choosing to augment their medical first-aid kits with a few homeopathic medicines. Arnica cream is particularly useful for bumps and bruises, and calendula cream is excellent for nappy rash and sore nipples in breast-feeding mothers. Chamomilla can offer babies relief from the pain of teething.

Training

The vast majority of professional homeopaths are self-employed in their own private practices. Some practitioners work independently, while others work in homeopathy centres or multidisciplinary clinics. Homeopaths have often trained full-time for two years or part-time for four years and have undergone one year's supervised clinical experience, in order to practise and to become a member of the homeopathy governing association of the country in which they practise.

Osteopathy

Osteopathy is based on treating the joints and muscles of the body, and it regards the body as a whole entity. It is most commonly used to treat problems in the back and neck, and joint complaints; however, it can be used to address most mobility and structural problems within the body. The methods used in osteopathy aim to increase mobility and reduce pain through natural, non-invasive manipulation of the body.

Osteopaths use conventional methods of diagnosis to assess the patient who has come to them, and then help to return the patient's body to its optimum condition without the use of drugs or surgery (which are retained as last-resort options).

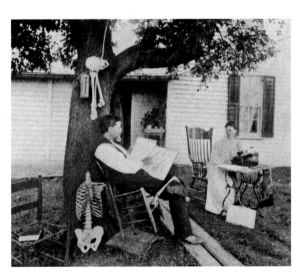

Left The American doctor Andrew Taylor Still founded osteopathy in the late 19th century.

Opposite *Osteopathy is used to increase mobility and reduce pain through gentle manipulation.*

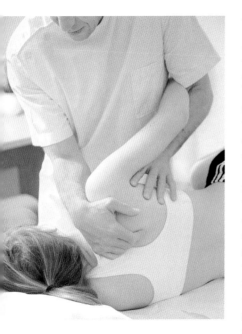

Who can benefit?

Many osteopathy sessions are a direct result of the patient seeking out an osteopath, rather than being referred by their physician (although some doctors do refer their patients to an osteopath, especially in cases where drugs or surgery are not necessary).

Osteopathy is commonly used for whiplash and similar injuries, where it can be difficult to diagnose the source and severity of an injury without the help of a specialist. Osteopaths also regularly treat sports complaints, ranging from muscle damage and trauma to simple muscle- and joint-strengthening. This therapy is also good as a preventative treatment for sportsmen and women – a practitioner can diagnose how and why an injury happened and offer a plan to avoid it in future. Problems such as poor technique, or excessive strain being placed upon certain areas of the body due to being overweight or under-strength, can also be recognized by an osteopath and planned for accordingly, by changing technique or tailoring an activity regime.

History

Osteopathy was founded in Kansas in 1874 by Andrew Taylor Still (1828–1917). He declared that the bone (osteon) was the primary point from which it was possible to diagnose the cause of pathological conditions, and thus named it osteopathy. The therapy came to the UK about a century ago, with the first practice opening in London in 1917.

Osteopaths frequently deal with pregnant women, as some of the symptoms of pregnancy affect the muscles and joints. Carrying an extra load can put a strain on your back and legs, so strengthening is important to prevent pain or problems occurring later in life. Osteopathy also helps with foot pain, posture, headaches, and stress, all of which can be symptoms of pregnancy. It can also be used on children and babies.

What to expect

Before you begin any osteopathy sessions, always check that your osteopath is registered with the governing association in your country of residence.

In the first instance the osteopath will try to establish some background, by going over your medical history and general health. He or she may also go over your family history and lifestyle, although this should not be necessary if the issue is an injury that was the result of an incident such as a sports trauma.

Next, the osteopath will try to establish the nature of the injury, and its severity, by diagnosing your symptoms and giving you a physical assessment. He or she will do this by examining your muscles and joints, possibly moving your joints and observing the movements. In more serious cases, or those that may be difficult to diagnose, the osteopath may arrange for an X-ray or MRI (magnetic resonance imaging)

CAUTION

If you have fractured bones, you should not seek the help of an osteopath, but should instead consult a doctor or emergency department. It is also inadvisable to seek treatment from an osteopath if you suffer from osteoporosis, cancer, or blood-clotting, and you should always check with your healthcare practitioner before seeing an osteopath under these circumstances; if he or she deems it to be safe and useful for you to see an osteopath, they will refer you to a registered practitioner.

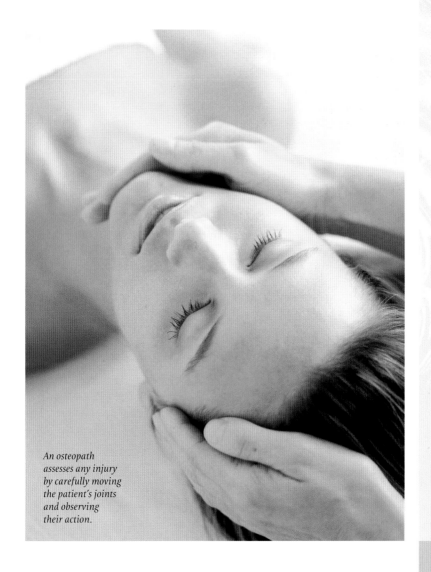

An osteopath assesses any injury by carefully moving the patient's joints and observing their action.

scan, or other forms of clinical observation. Once the cause of the problem has been identified, the osteopath will discuss treatment options with you, devising a treatment plan and detailing the number of sessions you will need; how they will treat the issue; and whether there are any factors in your life that should be changed, such as your lifestyle or sports technique. The level and length of treatment will depend on the injury, your medical and family history, and how long the issue has been troubling you.

Treatment involves the patient sitting or lying down on a table and the osteopath gently applying a carefully judged amount of manual pressure in one precise direction. He or she will either apply pressure directly to the area that is giving you problems or to an area close by. This technique is used to relax the tissues (put them at ease) or to engage them at their functional limit so that it can have an effect on structural and tissue abnormalities, relieve joint restriction and misalignment, restore balance in the muscles and tissue, and encourage the movement of bodily fluids.

Training

To become an osteopath, candidates usually have to complete a four- or five-year degree to gain either a bachelor's degree (a BSc with Honours, a BOst [Bachelor of Osteopathy], or a BOstMed) or a master's degree in osteopathy. In the UK the term "osteopath" is protected by law, and anyone caught practising without the correct qualifications or registration could face criminal charges. Similar laws apply in the US and other countries.

STUDY FACT

Osteopaths have a reputation for being able to diagnose when a patient is not suitable for osteopathic treatment. In this case they will refer you to a suitable doctor or specialist, in order for you to receive the most appropriate treatment.

Chiropractic

Chiropractic uses manipulation of the body to treat and prevent problems in the musculoskeletal system. These manipulative techniques are designed to relieve pain and improve the function of joints and muscle spasms, without the use of drugs or surgery.

They involve soft-tissue massage and stretching, spinal adjustments, and moving the joints – sometimes further than you would be able to achieve independently. This is done to normalize the function of the joints and to help alleviate pain.

Despite strong opposition when this therapy was first established, because many people believed that it was a way for charlatans to practise medicine without a licence, chiropractic has grown around the world and is now the third-largest healthcare profession globally.

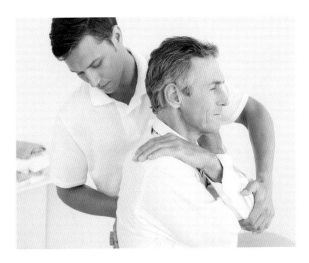

Spinal adjustment is an integral part of a chiropractic manipulation.

History

The practice of manipulating the body – and in particular the spine – to relieve pain and improve the musculoskeletal system has been around for centuries, having been performed in ancient Greek and Chinese civilizations. Chiropractic is named from the Greek words *cheir*, meaning "hands", and *praktos*, meaning "done". The modern practice was established in 1895 in Iowa by Daniel David Palmer (1845–1913).

Who can benefit?

Chiropractic helps a range of musculoskeletal problems, in particular back pain, and its methods are safe for people of all ages because it does not involve the use of drugs or surgery.

Chiropractors often work with pregnant women and the elderly due to the musculoskeletal problems associated with pregnancy and growing old. Chiropractic treatment can help alleviate back pain, aching and painful joints, and arthritis. It is also safe to use on children, because its methods are non-invasive and are modified to each person's needs. Chiropractors can even work with babies when birth causes trauma to a baby and spinal

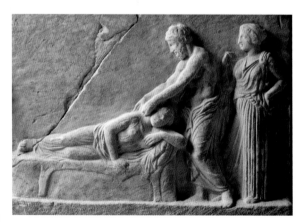

Left *The word "chiropractic" comes from the ancient Greek words "cheir" (hands) and "praktos" (done). Chiropractic was widely used in ancient Greece and China.*

Opposite *Modern founder, Daniel D Palmer, established chiropractic in 1895, opening a school two years later.*

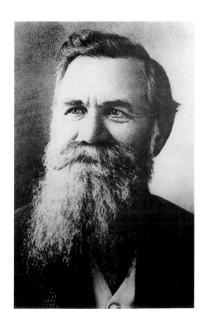

to establish the cause of your problem and to work out a plan and a timetable for treatment. The chiropractor will ask you to fill in a form about your medical history, and will then discuss this with you, as well as reviewing any medication that you may be taking and anything else that is relevant to the problem. If necessary, you may be taken for an X-ray or X-rayed on site if this facility exists.

Once the diagnosis is complete the chiropractor will go over the possible treatment options with you: discussing whether chiropractic is an appropriate treatment for you, what the treatment will involve, and outlining a timetable. After the options have been explained, and consent has been given, treatment may begin at that session.

During a typical chiropractic adjustment your chiropractor places you in specific positions to treat affected areas. Often you are positioned lying face-down on a padded table that is similar to a massage table. Using only his or her hands, the chiropractor will give the joint sudden, yet

or cranial misalignment could create problems in childhood and/or adulthood if left untreated.

You can seek the help of a private chiropractor or sometimes you may be referred by your physician or be able to seek treatment directly through your country's health service.

What to expect

At your first appointment with a chiropractor the aim will be

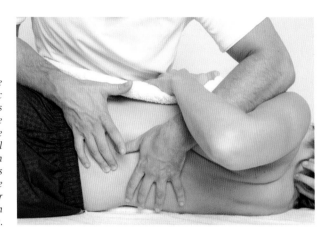

Many of the chiropractic adjustments centre on the spine and the client will be placed in specific positions to allow the chiropractor access with his hands.

controlled force that takes it beyond its normal range. Don't be concerned if you hear your joints popping or cracking during the treatment session – that is perfectly normal.

Other treatment approaches that are often recommended as being compatible with chiropractic adjustment range from heat or ice and massage and stretching to electrical stimulation, exercise, and/or weight loss.

After the chiropractic adjustment you may experience minor side-effects for a few days. These may include headache, fatigue, or pain in the parts of the body that have been treated.

Training

In the UK the term "chiropractor" is protected, and it is illegal to practise chiropractic without being a member of the General Chiropractic Council. Chiropractors are legally allowed to use the term "doctor" when they practise, as long as it is made clear that they are a doctor of chiropractic and not a medical practitioner. In order to become a registered chiropractor, candidates in most countries must complete a four-year chiropractic degree.

Hypnotherapy

Hypnotherapy is the process of entering a deep state of relaxation so that your mind will be more open to suggestion. In this state the hypnotherapist will help you to make positive changes in your life, which you may previously have been wary of or believed to be too difficult – or even impossible – to change.

Almost everyone has the potential to be hypnotized, although some people are more susceptible than others. The main factor in how easily someone can be hypnotized is how willing they are to undergo

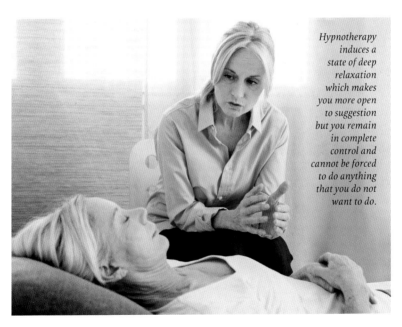

Hypnotherapy induces a state of deep relaxation which makes you more open to suggestion but you remain in complete control and cannot be forced to do anything that you do not want to do.

47

the process. If you do not wish to experience hypnosis then it will be very difficult for the hypnotherapist (or anyone, for that matter) to induce a deep, relaxed state. If you are willing, and have trust and confidence in the hypnotherapist, then it will be far easier to induce a relaxed state.

Some people are afraid of hypnosis because they think they will have no control and that they will be at the mercy of the hypnotherapist. This is a common misconception. While hypnotized, you remain in complete control and can even wake yourself up if there is a problem or you feel uncomfortable. You cannot be forced to do anything you do not want to do. Hypnosis is merely a way of making you more open to suggestion and not a way of forcing you to accept suggestion. (It is important to remember that stage acts, such as those seen in entertainment shows and on television, involve willing participants who consent to take part and are expecting to act foolishly or do whatever else is asked of them; and they could still refuse to do so, while hypnotized, if they wished.)

History

It is difficult to establish a definitive starting point for the hypnotherapy treatment with which we are familiar today. For centuries different cultures have used the practice of inducing a trance-like state when treating medical problems or seeking enlightenment. Shamans and witch doctors are believed to have used hypnosis when searching for an answer to a question. Many cultures also use drug-induced trances to achieve the same goals, and these are referred to as narcohypnosis-induced states.

The father of modern hypnotherapy was a Scottish doctor James Esdaile (1808–59) who was working as a surgeon in India during the 1830s when he first encountered hypnotism. At first he believed it to be a trick or a con used to scam people into believing they were seeing one man control the mind of another. However, after some experimentation of his own,

Dr Esdaile began to see the potential for the use of hypnosis in medicine. He went on to use it in thousands of his own operations, apparently including up to 19 amputations.

Who can benefit?

Although hypnotherapy is principally used to help conditions of the mind, advocates claim that it can also help alleviate physical ailments. And many people seek hypnotherapy for pain relief; it is becoming increasingly popular as a way to control labour pain without resorting to drugs, to reduce the length of labour and the need for interventions such as Caesarean sections. Nonetheless, the most common use of hypnotherapy is to affect behavioural changes, such as weight loss and addictions, phobias, and sexual disorders.

Hypnotherapy is safe for all ages, including children and the elderly, and for all conditions.

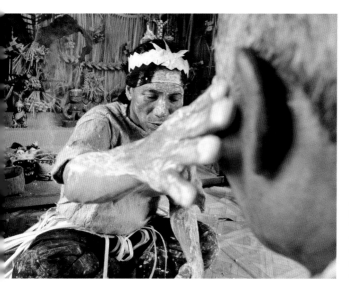

For centuries shaman have used hypnosis when treating medical issues or when seeking enlightenment.

However, any patient who could be considered vulnerable (such as a child or a patient with a carer) should be accompanied by a responsible adult at each session. When seeking hypnotherapy for treatment of a child, always ask the therapist what experience they have in dealing with children.

What to expect

In the first session the hypnotherapist will establish your history, what the problem is and its roots, and how to provide a solution. This is an opportunity to ask any questions you may have about the therapy, or about your practitioner, in order to put your mind at rest and establish a level of trust which will help you to become more relaxed in sessions and will increase the effectiveness of the therapy.

The hypnotherapist will relax you in a number of possible ways: by using music, asking you to lie or sit on a couch or seat, and talking to you in a calm way. Every practitioner uses a different approach. When you are in a deep relaxed state (trance), you may be asked to imagine a pleasant place where you feel comfortable, such as a beach or garden. You will be able to hear your hypnotherapist's voice throughout the treatment, and he or she will continue to talk to you to keep you relaxed and to deepen the trance so that you can access your subconscious mind more easily. The practitioner will then use the power of suggestion to attempt to alter your behaviour, your thinking, or your actions to resolve the problem.

CAUTION

Hypnotherapy should not be used to deal with serious mental conditions such as schizophrenia or dementia, nor should it be used if you suffer from epilepsy, narcolepsy, or serious heart conditions.

A hypnotherapist may use various methods to relax you, including playing music and talking to you as you sit or lie down.

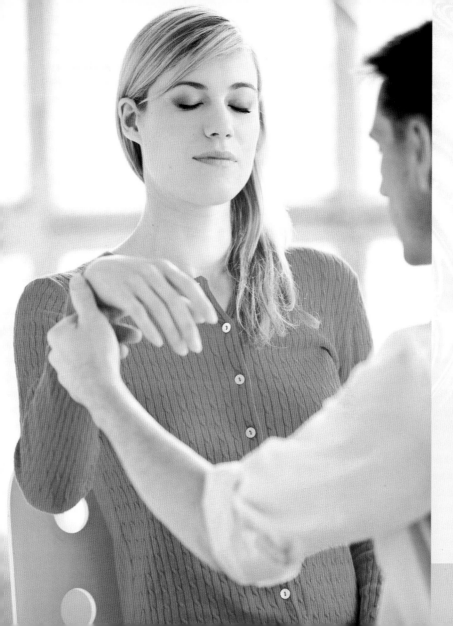

Once you are brought out of your trance you will feel re-energized. The hypnotherapist may give you a hypnotherapy CD or may teach you methods for relaxation at home. These are not a substitute for professional help, but rather a method of reinforcing and complementing the work that has been done with your practitioner, and they will help your therapy to progress.

Training

As hypnotherapy is not regulated in some countries (including the UK), it is not a legal requirement to undergo any sort of training to become a hypnotherapist, so it is very important to see a practitioner who is registered with the accredited organizations.

STUDY FACT

For hypnotherapy to have the optimum effect as a method of pain-control during labour, it is recommended that treatment start around week 32 of pregnancy.

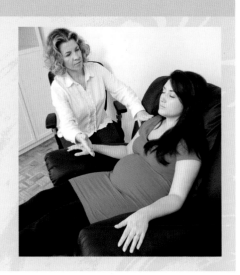

Hypnotherapists offering hypnosis for labour and birth do not promise a pain-free experience but say that many women who give birth under hypnosis feel only discomfort and a sensation of pressure through labour and even through delivery.

Herbal medicine

Herbs have been used as the primary form of medicine for centuries. Almost all civilizations and cultures over the millennia have used natural organic remedies from their surrounding ecosystems. It is the original and oldest form of medicine, and its popularity has grown in recent years as different plants, herbs, and methods have been discovered, shared, and transported all over the world.

A new generation of herbs and their components are now being discovered and explored for their healing properties, and it is an exciting time in herbal medicine.

Herbs can be used to treat a wide range of ailments in a variety of different forms, ranging from creams, oils, and balms to tablets, teas, and leaves for chewing.

Herbal medicine is incredibly hard to regulate. No licence is required to administer herbal remedies, and the only regulation that has been implemented is the

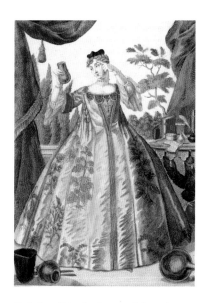

Herbal medicine has been used throughout history and was at the height of its popularity from the Middle Ages until the advent of modern medicine in the 19th century.

formation of a central agency responsible for testing the safety and quality of all available herbal remedies (see the box on page 56). You are advised to choose a practitioner who is registered with one of the governing associations.

Who can benefit?

Herbal remedies can be used to treat a great many ailments, and they are particularly effective at treating:

- Problems of the immune system and autoimmune conditions
- Allergies
- Chronic fatigue syndrome
- Hormonal health
- Fertility
- Digestion
- Emotional health
- Skin conditions
- Joint and bone problems.

People with chronic conditions, and those with problems that have no actual cure, often consult herbalists, who can alleviate their symptoms effectively. For example, the menopause and irritable bowel syndrome (IBS) are among the most common complaints that have no cure, but which herbal remedies can help to alleviate.

What to expect

All herbal remedies available for purchase over the counter come with clear instructions for

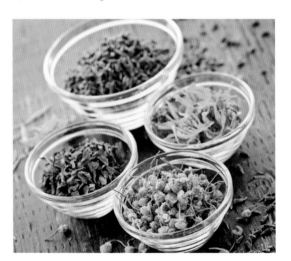

Left *An experienced herbal medicine practitioner will combine various plants into a treatment that is tailored specifically for your situation.*

Opposite *Medicinal herb charts show a picture of the plant together with either its common or Latin name. Some will even list the properties and actions of each plant.*

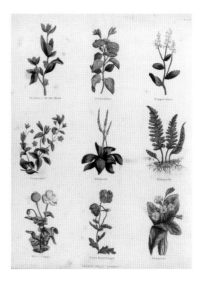

application. If you visit a herbal practitioner you should first check the type of therapy that he or she offers and whether it is suitable for your particular condition, because there is a wide range of treatments and herbalists often specialize.

Once you have found a practitioner who is right for you, the first session will familiarize your practitioner with your situation. This will involve a full medical examination (which may include blood and/or urine tests),

CAUTION

Although people of all ages have been using herbal medicine for centuries, market-wide licensing and registration are still relatively new, and the safety of herbal medicine for some groups of the population – including children and the elderly – has not yet been established. Pregnant women and breast-feeding mothers should be aware that the chemicals from herbal medicines may be absorbed by the foetus or breast-feeding child.

Herbal remedies can also interact with other medicines, and if you are being prescribed medicines, or have ever suffered from kidney or liver problems, you should always consult your physician before taking herbal treatments. Similarly, if you suffer from any serious medical conditions, always talk to your healthcare practitioner before pursuing any alternative therapies.

questions about your own and your family's medical history, and about your lifestyle, diet, and problem. The practitioner will then go on to assemble an individual treatment plan or prescription for you, explaining the timeline for your treatment and any instructions that you may need.

Once the treatment – which may take the form of herbal decoctions, syrups, tinctures, teas, or infused oils, salves, ointments, and creams – is complete, the herbalist will arrange a follow-up session with you, in order to assess your recovery. You will be asked questions about your condition, how you are progressing, and any problems with the treatment that you are encountering. If necessary, the herbalist will make adjustments to your treatment.

Training

The Medicines and Healthcare Products Regulatory Agency (MHRA) governs the use of herbal

INDUSTRY REGULATION

Herbal products have been unlicensed for years, but in the UK the MHRA has gradually phased out unlicensed products and is responsible for the quality assessment of products and devices released into the country. In the US the FDA, and in Europe the European Medicines Agency, performs a similar task.

As of April 2011, products in Europe (including the UK) must have a traditional herbal registration or a product licence. Licensed remedies are tested to the same standards as all medicine, ensuring that they are safe, reliable, and have instructions for use.

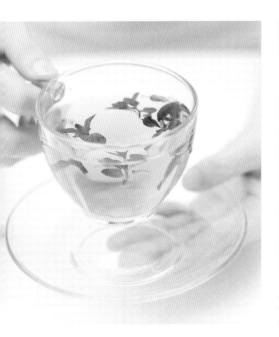

STUDY FACT

If you are planning to claim herbal treatment through private insurance, you should always check with your insurance company that herbal medicine is included in your insurance plan, and whether you need to be referred by a physician.

Herbal remedies can be used in various forms, from ointments and oils to tinctures and teas.

remedies in the UK, just as the Food and Drug Administration (FDA) does in the US. Practitioners must meet the minimum requirements for safe and effective practice, with ongoing professional development. They can also choose to become part of a professional body such as the National Institute of Medical Herbalists in the UK, the European Herbal and Traditional Medicine Practitioners Association, and the American Herbalists Guild. In the US practitioners must be licensed as naturopathic doctors or acupuncturists to be able to diagnose and practise legally; they often study as interns with experienced herbalists before setting up their own practices.

Reiki

Reiki is a method of natural healing that focuses on the use of universal life force/energy to restore health and well-being. Reiki energy is regarded as life energy at its most effective – with maximum vibration. Reiki is one of the fastest-growing healing therapies currently being taught.

According to Eastern traditions, all parts of us – body, mind, emotions, and spirit – need to be in harmony in order to be truly healthy. The pressures of modern life can result in our personal energy (*qi*) running low, which in turn can lead to a suppressed immune system, leaving us vulnerable to sickness and pain, and to emotional and mental-health problems.

A reiki practitioner is a conduit for the reiki energy, reconnecting the recipient to the universal life energy. The energy is channelled through the therapist's hands, which are placed on the body or just over the body, generally in

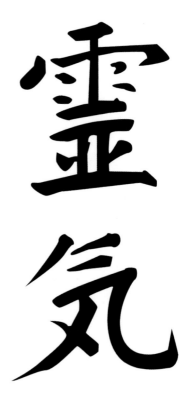

The word 'reiki' in Japanese calligraphy. The top kanji, 'rei', means 'spirit or soul' and the bottom kanji, 'ki', means 'life force'.

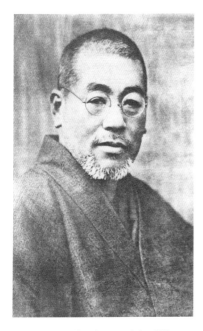

Dr Mikao Usui first discovered the ability to transfer healing reiki energy in 1922.

History

Reiki (pronounced "ray-key") is Japanese for "universal life energy". It was first discovered by Dr Mikao Usui (1865–1926), a Japanese theologist who perfected the ability to transfer reiki energy in 1922. He then taught others how to act as channels for this energy. Every reiki practitioner can trace their professional heritage back to Dr Usui.

Who can benefit?

Reiki can be used for general well-being and to restore the body's energy flow. It is also useful for:

• Pain relief
• Relaxation
• Stress relief
• Emotional relief
• Aiding sleep
• Improving energy levels
• Calming excitable children
• Pregnancy and labour.

It works on the principle of knowing where universal energy needs to go, rather than on the practitioner's diagnosis. As such, reiki healing can be used

positions corresponding to the seven major chakras (or energy centres, see page 176) of the body. Some experienced reiki practitioners and reiki masters use their intuition when it comes to the placing of the hands, saying that they are drawn to the areas that are in most need of healing.

effectively on household pets, animals, and even plants.

What to expect

As the practitioner will want to familiarize himself or herself with you on your first visit, this may take a little longer than a normal session. Appointments usually last in the region of 45–90 minutes.

You will remain fully clothed throughout the treatment and will usually lie on a couch, although reiki can also be given while seated if you have mobility problems or are elderly. Often relaxing music is played and the lighting is dim or candle-lit.

Once the practitioner is ready, having followed their own specific preparation routine, he or she will start by placing the hands over various parts of your body. Some therapists use a light touch, while others hover their hands just above the body, without making any physical contact. Reiki is a whole-body treatment because practitioners believe that no single part of the body exists in isolation, and that disease or disorder in one area

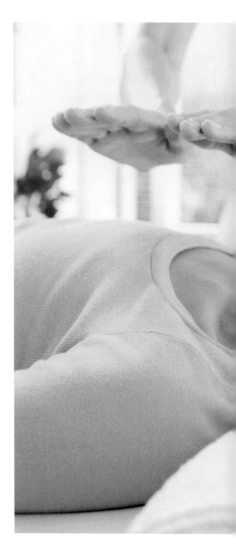

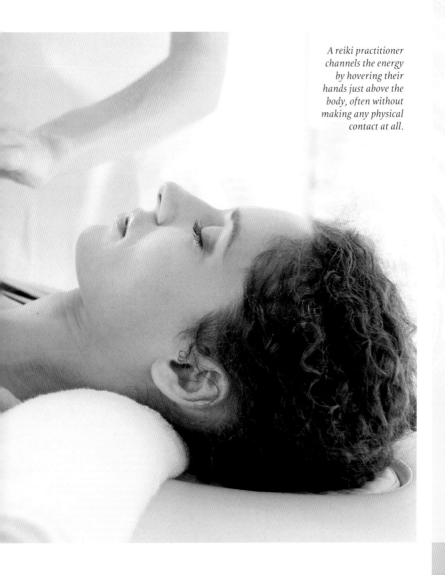

A reiki practitioner channels the energy by hovering their hands just above the body, often without making any physical contact at all.

HIGHER LEVELS

The highest form of reiki is reiki-do, also known as "the way of reiki" or "the path of universal life energy". It follows the same principles as reiki, but is used principally for personal growth and as a way to live life. The three categories of reiki-do are "inner work" (based on meditation), "outer work" (using reiki energy with chakras, crystals, and other therapies), and "synergistic work" (a merger of inner and outer reiki-do, where the effect is greater than the sum of its parts).

Over a period of time, and with regular whole-body sessions, the body's energy channels are opened to allow it to deal effectively with stress and any build-up of toxins, and general well-being is restored. Reiki therapy can also provide the necessary energy to aid recovery from illness and is a useful complementary therapy to other modalities.

Training

There are three levels of training in order to become a reiki master: the first, second, and master degrees. At each degree the trainee receives attunements (the process whereby the ability to give reiki treatments is transmitted via the master teacher) from the reiki energy. After each attunement the higher vibrations of reiki energy will join the trainee's energy field.

Once the first-degree level has been passed the trainee is able to use reiki to heal himself or herself and others. Physical healing is the first rung on the reiki ladder. At second-degree level, the "keys" or "symbols" to help heal on

will inevitably have an effect on the rest of the body.

You may feel warmth or a tingling sensation as the practitioner works through a sequence of movements. Most people report feeling extremely relaxed after a reiki session. Do make sure that you drink plenty of water following treatment to help the detoxification process.

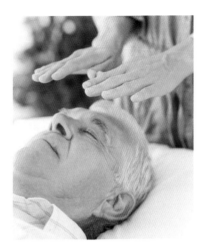

Most people report feeling extremely relaxed after a reiki treatment, which is why it is so popular as an effective treatment for stress.

an emotional and mental level are taught. Distance healing (sending healing to those who are geographically distant from you) is also taught.

The third degree takes the trainee to master level, where the practitioner is qualified not only to take responsibility for his or her own healing, but also to help others deal with their soul issues. They also learn how to pass attunements to teach, or "attune", others to reiki.

SEICHEM

Seichem (which is pronounced "*say-keem*") is a very similar treatment to reiki, but instead of placing the hands on the body the practitioner works in the aura surrounding the body. It is believed that the ancient Egyptians may well have practised the healing art of Seichem. According to its tenets, there are four elemental rays – namely, earth, water, air, and fire – of which reiki is one (earth).

While visiting Egypt in 1980, Patrick Zeigler spent a night in the King's Chamber of the Great Pyramid, and it was here that he rediscovered Seichem. This therapy connects with your higher self, so that healing can take place in the physical, mental, emotional, and spiritual bodies. The therapy uses energy to heal, but also to stimulate personal development and growth. Although the spelling of the word may differ, its meaning is always "power" in the spiritual sense of the word.

Reflexology

Reflexology is an ancient therapy involving the gentle manipulation of the feet (or occasionally the hands or ears) to stimulate the body's own healing process. Its underlying principle is similar to that of acupuncture (see page 18), in that each pressure point on the sole or sides of the foot (hand or ear) corresponds to a particular function or part of the body.

However, the meridian lines or zones of the body are described differently in reflexology from those used in acupuncture. Every organ and system of the body has a corresponding "reflex point" on the foot (hand or ear) and, by applying pressure to these specific points, the corresponding part of the body is stimulated to improve its functioning and to get rid of toxins, thereby allowing the body to heal itself.

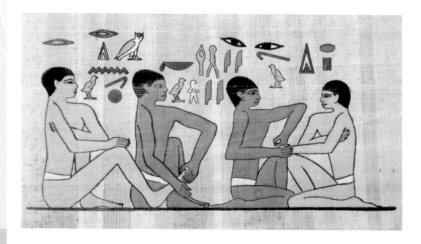

History

Although reflexology dates back to ancient China and ancient Egypt, it was Dr William Fitzgerald (see the box, right) who revived the principle in the early 20th century. He applied pressure to parts of the foot and discovered that it anaesthetized corresponding parts of the body. He called this system Zone Therapy, and it became the forerunner of what we know today as reflexology.

And it was a nurse and physiotherapist called Eunice

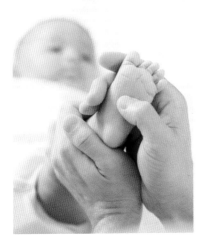

Opposite *An early reference to reflexology in an Ancient Egyptian tomb shows the official Ptahhotep (c. 2465–2325 BCE) having his hands, feet, and legs massaged by a servant.*

Left *Babies respond well to reflexology as their feet have undeveloped arches, and the skin and bones are quite soft. Gently rubbing the feet can release blockages and restore energy flow, soothing cranky babies and helping to relieve tummy pains.*

Ingham (1889–1974) who first pioneered the form of reflexology that we now recognize, and who produced a map of the entire body relating to specific reflex points on the feet.

Who can benefit?

Reflexology is suitable for a wide range of conditions, but is particularly appropriate for any circulation or stress-related problems. It has also been used

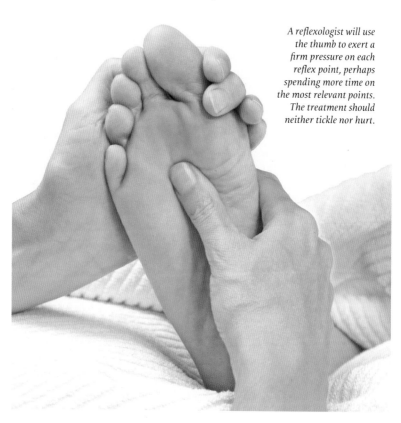

A reflexologist will use the thumb to exert a firm pressure on each reflex point, perhaps spending more time on the most relevant points. The treatment should neither tickle nor hurt.

successfully in the treatment of fertility issues. There is currently medical interest in reflexology for pain management in the chronically ill, and it has become a popular choice for pain relief during pregnancy and labour. Although there is no scientific explanation for reflexology, doctors are gradually becoming more accepting of this therapy.

The only barrier to treating infants is the size of their feet. For this reason reflexology tends to be most suitable for toddlers over the age of one or two. However, reflexologists claim a good success rate in treating childhood problems such as hyperactivity and "glue ear".

What to expect

Reflexology looks at the underlying causes for symptoms, so your initial treatment will probably address you as a whole, rather than solely your specific ailment. A thorough consultation – involving your full medical history and aspects of your lifestyle and well-being – means that the first session is longer than most, taking a full hour and a half, whereas follow-up treatments will last for around 45–60 minutes.

Reflexology is a non-invasive therapy and you will merely be asked to take off your shoes and socks. The treatment should be relaxing. The therapist exerts firm pressure with the thumb on each reflex point, working from the toes towards the ankle. You may occasionally experience some pricking pain in the foot when a particularly sensitive area is being worked on, but, contrary to popular belief, reflexology does not tickle. Some practitioners use creams or oils to aid massage, while others work directly on the skin. You will be encouraged to drink water after the treatment, to help flush toxins from your system.

Some people experience a slight reaction to treatment the following day – perhaps mild flu-like symptoms, a slight skin rash, or you might feel emotional. This is a sign that the body is beginning to detoxify and heal itself, and the symptoms should pass fairly quickly. Another common side-effect is more

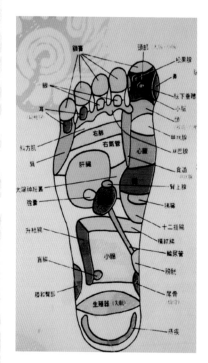

頭部
腦垂腺
鼻
腦下垂體
小腦
頸
曲頭腺
淋巴腺
右肺
右氣管
心臟
食道
肝臟
腎上腺
腎臟
十二指腸
橫結腸
輸尿管
膀胱
尾骨
生殖器 (大腿)
痔疾
額竇
眼
耳
斜方肌
肩
大溫神經叢
脊柱
升結腸
盲腸
小腸
骶和臀部

Foot reflexology charts show the location of reflex points on the feet. The charts are based on zones that reflect the body in miniature on our feet.

frequent urination following a treatment. Weekly reflexology sessions are recommended, usually for about six weeks, depending on your condition.

Training

Those who want to make a career of being a reflexologist need to make sure their qualification is widely recognized and offers them insurance and professional back-up, leading to membership of the professional association in their country. It is worth noting that there is no protection of the title of reflexologist in some countries (including the UK), so anyone can call themselves a reflexologist.

If you simply want to treat friends and family, then countless reflexology courses are available, and insurance and professional support are not an issue. Bear in mind that distance learning is not a good idea for manual therapies, because you need to feel in person what you are learning.

Nutritional therapy

Nutritional therapy uses nutritional science to help people to stay healthy, to achieve peak performance, and for individual care. A registered nutritional therapist is trained to spot and assess any nutritional imbalances using a wide range of tools, and to work out what part these imbalances play in your symptoms and health concerns. It is their job to work alongside you in establishing a better nutritional balance and in finding ways to help you maintain a healthy body using a programme that is specifically tailored to your personal needs, rather than a "one size fits all" approach.

Who can benefit?

Increasingly, people are turning to nutritional therapists when they are faced with a chronic health problem that conventional medicine is unable to treat. Such problems range from allergies, digestive and bowel disorders, hormonal imbalances, and fatigue to depression or stress, autoimmune conditions, migraine, and skin disorders. Children with learning and behavioural difficulties, as well as overweight children, often benefit from support with nutritional therapy.

A growing number of people now have an allergic reaction to certain foods, although they may not realize that this is the cause of any number of chronic ailments. Nutritional therapy is excellent for detecting and dealing with this hidden cause. Research also shows that junk-food diets are associated with antisocial behaviour, and that nutritional therapy can dramatically improve the disposition of young offenders and difficult school children, by giving them better food and supplements. If you adopt a nutritional and lifestyle approach to your health, it has been shown that all the major systems of the body can benefit.

Typically, a nutritional therapist will emphasize the importance of trying to reach optimum energy levels, achieve a good blood-sugar balance, aim for emotional and psychological well-being, and optimize gastrointestinal health so that you can tolerate a broad range of food groups.

What to expect

At your first consultation the practitioner will almost certainly ask you to fill in a health and nutrition questionnaire. You will also be asked for details about your personal health, medical and family history, and your lifestyle choices, and typically this session will last 60–90 minutes. Once the practitioner has evaluated your particular needs, she or he will tailor-make a programme of nutritional and lifestyle changes that are safe, effective, and unique to you.

You should expect to go back for a follow-up appointment around four weeks later to check on your progress and to make any necessary adjustments. Depending on how well the programme suits you, there may be the need for further consultations.

Training

Make sure that the nutritional practitioner you choose is fully qualified – whichever country you live in, ensure that the therapist you have chosen belongs to a professional association.

CAUTION

Nutritional therapy is not a replacement for medical advice, and a nutritional practitioner will always refer any client with "red flag" signs or symptoms to the medical profession. Nutritional therapists often work alongside medical professionals and are usually happy to explain any nutritional-therapy programme that has been provided.

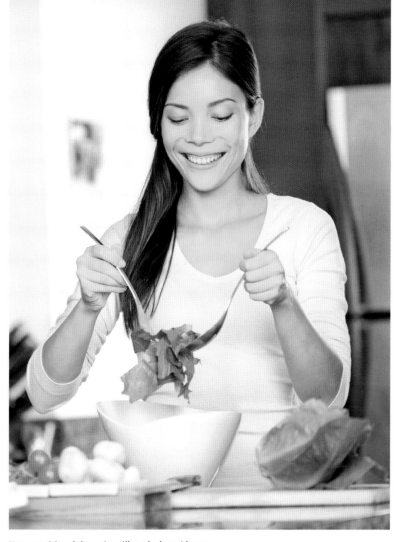

Your nutritional therapist will work alongside you to help you establish a better nutritional balance.

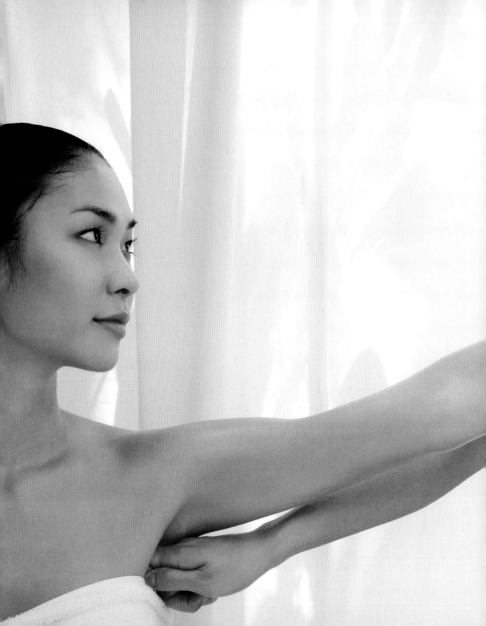

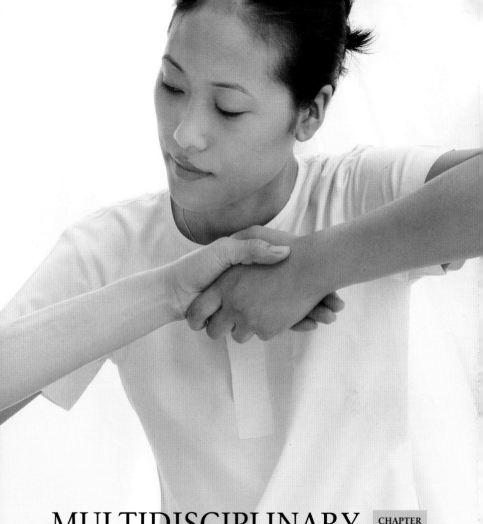

MULTIDISCIPLINARY HEALING SYSTEMS

Ayurveda

Ayurveda means "the science of life" in Sanskrit. According to Ayurvedic principles, 107 marma points (see also pages 28–9) on the body govern our muscular, skeletal, and nervous systems. The mind has considerable influence on the body and, in keeping with other great systems of medicine, the concept of balancing the energies or life forces to achieve harmony of mind and body is central to Ayurvedic philosophy.

The emphasis is placed on individuality. The human body has three distinct kinds of energy forces, or *doshas*: Vata governs our nervous and circulatory systems, Kapha governs our cells and structure, and Pitta governs our metabolism. If these three forces

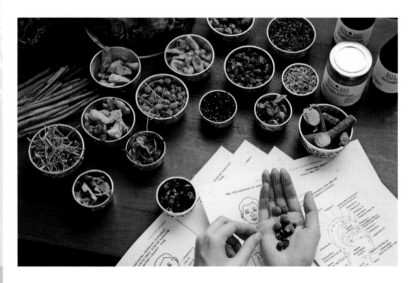

stay in balance, then we remain healthy; but if one or more *dosha* is out of balance – perhaps caused by poor diet, the environment, or our mental state – then we become ill.

Ayurveda offers you a journey to well-being. You have to let go and trust in the process – it is not a quick fix. A consultation will show you where you are: physically, energetically, mentally, and emotionally.

History

Ayurvedic medicine is a holistic system that was first practised in India long before the ancient Greeks or the Chinese developed their own healing philosophies. Vedic scriptures recorded in Sanskrit 5,000 years ago show that an intellectual and spiritually advanced culture existed in human society, which covered philosophy, architecture,

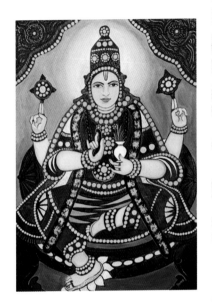

Opposite *An Ayurvedic practitioner will almost certainly prescribe a herbal remedy for you alongside other treatments and dietary advice.*

Right *Vedic astrology is an integral part of a diagnosis in the Ayurvedic system.*

technical, cultural, political, medical, and astrological areas. However, it is the Ayurvedic treatments that translate into healing the body.

Who can benefit?

Ayurveda is largely used as a preventative medicine, but it can treat any illness (except for conditions that require surgery) and is particularly successful with chronic disorders that defy conventional medicine.

Allergy-based disorders, such as asthma, hay fever, migraines, and eczema, may be treated with a detoxification programme (known as *panchakarma*), herbal medicine, and yoga exercises. And marma massage is good for helping the recovery of stroke victims.

What to expect

Diagnosis takes the form of very close observation to determine your *dosha* or energy type, together with an examination of your Ayurvedic pulses. You will be asked about your lifestyle, family, and health problems. Your tongue and the colour of your skin and eyes may also be inspected.

Based on this information – together with your date, time, and

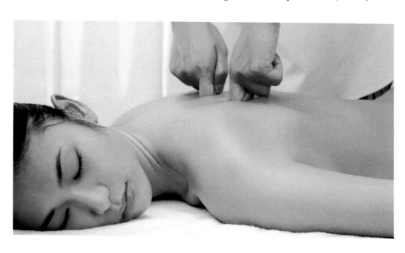

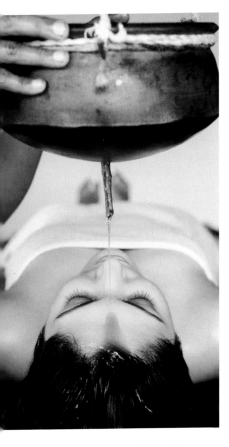

place of birth – your practitioner will quickly be able to establish which state (Vata, Pitta, or Kapha) you are currently in. By combining Vedic astrology (see the box on page 78) and Vedic medicine, the therapist will be able to assess you as a whole human being. From your chart, your pulse readings, and your answers to the medical questions, the therapist will then work out what herbs and tinctures you should be taking and will make them up for you. You will almost certainly also be given advice on your diet.

An Ayurvedic practitioner may well offer you marma-massage therapy. As we have seen, there are 107 marma points through which *prana*, or life force, flows by means of subtle channels of the body, including the seven chakras (or energy centres, see page 176) that are junctions between the physical body and the energetic body. Based on your pulse, your practitioner will decide which points to treat, and will then gently massage these, perhaps having selected specific

Above *Oils containing a blend of relevant essential oils may be used during a marma massage treatment.*

Opposite *Marma massage works through stimulating the body and massaging the 107 marma points (vital points).*

essential oils to apply very gently to these points.

Your practitioner may also recommend exercise in the form of yoga. The link between Ayurveda and yoga has a long history, and many scholars believe that you should always practise the two hand-in-hand – they have been linked sciences since the beginning, in ancient India. Between them, they

VEDIC ASTROLOGY

Vedic astrology is much older than Western astrology. It dates back thousands of years, whereas Western astrology is traceable only back to the millennium before Christ. Vedic astrology is primarily used to understand yourself and your karma (the sum of your actions) in this life.

The basic principle of Vedic astrology is that all things are linked. You are born when and where you are meant to be born, when everything is perfect for your incarnation, and your karmic experiences and your life are a reflection of the bigger picture into which you are born. Your Vedic chart will probably reflect your real life and your *dashas*: the predictive timelines that are used to predict when events will unfold in your life. *Dashas* offer a greater predictive accuracy than Western astrology. Vedic astrology tends to be less limited to talking about a general picture and can go much more deeply into what is going on in your life.

In Vedic astrology the 12 areas of your chart are the different departments of your life and are called *bhava*, which means "a way of being" or a "mood", and somehow sums everything up better. In Sanskrit, planets are called *graha*, which means "something that grasps". The planets are supposed to be the operators of karma, so they are holding you and directing what is happening in your life. That is how karma connects with your whole birth chart.

comprise a whole system of human development, in which yoga is the more spiritually orientated practice, while Ayurveda deals with therapy and treatment for the physical body as well as the mind. The interface between self-healing and self-realization is the union between yoga and Ayurveda.

Although these practices have diverged over the last 150 years, particularly in the West (where yoga without Ayurveda was for a long time considered normal), they are now being reintegrated. This synergy offers the harmonization of consciousness, life, healing, and transformation, and can help us to heal ourselves and our world, nature, mind, and spirit.

Training

For a list of accredited Ayurvedic practitioners you should consult the relevant professional body in your own country.

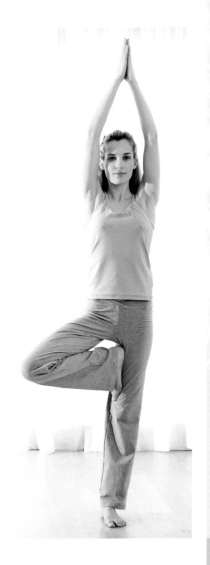

There is a traditional link between yoga and Ayurveda but exercise in general may be recommended by your practitioner.

Traditional Chinese Medicine

Traditional Chinese Medicine (TCM) is an ancient, all-encompassing system of healthcare that takes into account every aspect of the way we live, and treats each patient as an individual. After diagnosis, a number of different therapies – including acupuncture (see page 18), Chinese herbal medicine (see the box on page 84), tui na massage (see page 135), and preventative medicine (qigong exercise, see page 125, breathing techniques, diet, and lifestyle education) – are used to restore good health.

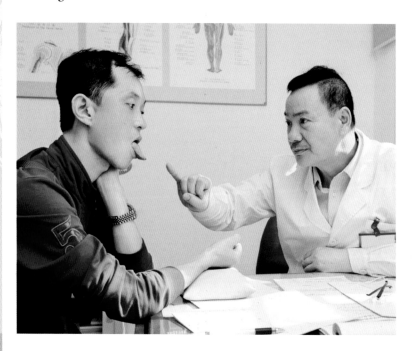

According to Chinese medicine, *qi* or energy flow through the body is the main determinant of our physical and mental well-being. Too much or too little activity in one or more of the 12 meridians (energy channels) is believed to be the cause of illness.

In the modern-day practice of TCM, the emphasis is placed firmly on restoring and maintaining harmony and balance in order to achieve good health, and on recognizing the link between the mind and the body. Two opposing forces regulate our moods and our health: Yin – the passive force; and Yang – the active force. The five basic elements of Chinese philosophy (fire, water, earth, matter, and wood) also play a vital role in our well-being and are crucial aids to diagnosis. According to this system of

Opposite The appearance of your tongue is an important factor during a TCM diagnosis.

Right Our well-being and physical/ emotional make-up are influenced by the five basic elements of fire, water, earth, matter, and wood.

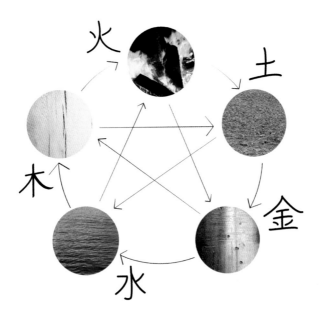

medicine, the heart, for instance, is a fire organ, while the kidney is a water organ. The organs of the body cooperate in complex ways, with implications for our emotions. If these functions get out of balance, illness is the result.

Symptoms are often described using the terms "hot", "cold", "damp", and so on, in various combinations. For example, too much stress in your life affects your liver, which then produces too much "fire" in your system and thus an imbalance.

History

TCM is a highly profound philosophy that is completely different from Western medical thinking, and it has had an uninterrupted history of development in China and other parts of East Asia dating back thousands of years.

Who can benefit?

In theory, any complaint and a person of any age can be treated by TCM, because all illness is caused by imbalance and TCM is a complete system of medicine. A combination of its integral therapies is used to treat illness, with Chinese herbs reputed to be especially beneficial for skin conditions, and acupuncture for back and neck pain, migraines, and headaches.

What to expect

A TCM practitioner will ask you about every aspect of your health and life, and will look very closely at your tastes, physical appearance, colouring, and even your personality. Your tongue will be examined for colour, shape, and condition. The

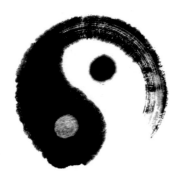

Our moods and our health are regulated by the opposing yet complementary forces of Yin (passive) and Yang (active).

practitioner will also check your wrists for pulse diagnosis.

Diagnosis of the underlying cause of your symptoms dictates the treatments that you might receive. That is why six people who apparently have the same condition may find themselves being treated in six different ways. Western doctors are still somewhat suspicious of TCM, although some are beginning to accept certain elements of it – acupuncture in particular.

Treatment times vary widely, depending on the therapies chosen and the severity of the case. Contrary to received Western wisdom, a chronic condition (such as weak energy) may warrant acupuncture treatment for an hour, while an acute pain (but with strong energy) may only warrant five minutes of treatment to stimulate healing.

Training

In ancient times Chinese doctors qualified by learning from their fathers, or from a master. However, in about 443 CE the Emperor started a college to train doctors in Chinese medicine. Some TCM practitioners still follow the family path, while others attend college to obtain their qualifications, although the resulting degree is not of relevance in all countries.

PREVENTATIVE MEDICINE

The philosophy of TCM puts great emphasis on preventative medicine. Practitioners will give educational training in how to know your body, and instruction in the ancient Chinese exercise system known as qigong (see page 125) or chi kung. Qigong offers a series of exercises, positions, and breathing techniques aimed at integrating the mind and body. The exercises, which relate to the acupuncture points on the body, are designed to stimulate the meridians or channels through which energy flows and to restore the balance of the body.

CHINESE HERBAL MEDICINE

According to the Australian Acupuncture and Chinese Medicine Association, "there are now more than 450 substances commonly used in Chinese herbal medicine – most are of plant origin, though some animal and mineral substances may also be used . . . Some substances that were used traditionally are no longer part of modern professional Chinese herbal medicine practice. For example, traditional remedies that are derived from endangered species have been replaced by other substances with similar actions."

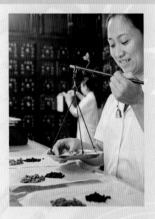

You may be prescribed a single herbal medicine, or it may be made into a formula, depending on whether or not you need the individual therapeutic action of one herb or would benefit more from a combined effect.

Herbal medicine may be prescribed singly or combined into a formula specifically tailored to your needs.

Sometimes herbs are prescribed in combination, so that any unwanted effects from an individual herb can be counteracted by the others in the formula.

Many people use TCM as a preventative medicine or to maintain general good health, but it also has a reputation for treating a wide range of health disorders, including:

- Insomnia
- Digestive disorders
- IBS
- Skin disorders
- Allergies
- Women's health problems (fertility, menstruation, and the menopause).

Naturopathy

Naturopathy is often described as the Western equivalent of Ayurveda or TCM, in that it is a distinct and total philosophy for life and health, which looks at the individual rather than the symptoms.

Its principles – namely, that the body has the power to heal and correct itself, and that illness is a reaction to disharmony and imbalance – were first established by Hippocrates in ancient Greece in around 400 BCE. If there is dysfunction in any area of the triad of health (the connection and interaction between the structural, biochemical, and mental/emotional components of all living beings), then there will be disruption or illness elsewhere. Moreover, the natural process of healing and recovery will bring back good health so long as nothing else interferes; and in modern terms, that includes drug treatments, which naturopaths believe can suppress symptoms

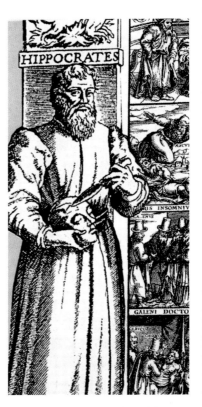

In 400 BCE, Hippocrates established that the body has the power to heal itself; naturopathy follows this principle.

and cause even worse problems to manifest at a later date.

Naturopaths seek to treat and avert disease or illness by bolstering the body's defence system, primarily through a nourishing diet, clean water, fresh air, and sunlight, as well as by means of appropriate exercise, rest, and relaxation. Many naturopaths also incorporate other therapeutic treatments, such as fasting (detoxification), acupressure or acupuncture, hydrotherapy (including colonic hydrotherapy; see the box on page 88), homeopathy, osteopathy, chiropractic, kinesiology, massage therapy, and herbal medicine. All these additional therapies share the basic principle of restoring the body's ability to self-correct, and maintain, a homeostatic balance and energy.

Naturopaths believe that we must all take responsibility for our own health. They place equal importance on educating and cooperating with you as they do on treating you.

Who can benefit?

Anyone with digestive problems, skin disorders, arthritic conditions, allergies, asthma, and hormonal problems will find that their conditions respond particularly well to the naturopathic approach. It is also excellent as a preventative health approach for all ages.

What to expect

A naturopathic practitioner will take an extremely detailed case-history on your first visit, covering not only your medical history and your actual complaint, but also your eating habits, the type of work you do, and your relationships. While many naturopaths use iris analysis

STUDY FACT

Naturopaths believe that a fever or diarrhoea is a sign that the body is fighting and shaking off an infection or an intrusion.

(see Iridology on page 180) as part of their diagnosis, others use medical techniques such as X-rays, blood tests, and urine tests as well.

Once a diagnosis has been made, the naturopath will advise you on diet, exercise, and any other recommended treatment. In general, naturopaths regard a balanced, organic, and partly raw-food diet (possibly involving fasting) as the best form of medicine; some also use treatments such as acupuncture, colonic hydrotherapy, and herbal or homeopathic remedies as a way of stimulating the body's energy to restore homeostasis (equilibrium), but definitely not to suppress

Iris analysis is just one of the diagnostic tools used by a naturopath.

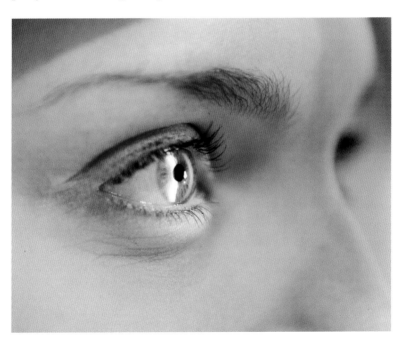

symptoms. Many naturopaths are also osteopaths, so you might receive massage or manipulation as part of your treatment.

As an example of a treatment plan, if you were suffering from rheumatoid arthritis, you might be advised to reduce your intake of protein, and be given poultices and water treatment for your inflamed joints.

Follow-up sessions to check on your progress usually take place once every two weeks. Chronic conditions take longer to get results than acute conditions. Don't be alarmed if you have a "healing crisis" shortly after your treatment commences – symptoms may recur from time to time as the body's energy returns. Naturopathic treatments encourage the body's natural immunity, and this may manifest itself in inflammation and fever.

Training

Qualified naturopaths have often completed a four-year full-time course, or a postgraduate course; you can check with the professional association of your own country to find a qualified naturopath practising near you.

COLONIC HYDROTHERAPY

This therapy involves flushing waste material out of the bowel, using water. You will be invited to lie on your side, and then a tube will be inserted into your back passage, through which water will start to flow. Waste products are flushed out of your body as the water circulates through your colon. Expect the procedure to last somewhere in the region of 30–40 minutes. Remarkably, around 60l (105pt) of water will have been introduced into your body during that time. Sometimes herbal infusions are added to the water for additional benefit.

CAUSES OF ILLNESS

The causes of the disease take primacy over the symptoms, for a naturopath. It is the causes that they want to identify and remove, whether these are chemical, mechanical, or psychological.

- **CHEMICAL CAUSES:** Naturopaths will take a close look at your diet, what you drink, and the air you breathe, as well as the organs of elimination, which include the bowels, kidneys, skin, and lungs. Any imbalance between these factors can lead to illness.

- **MECHANICAL CAUSES:** A naturopath is also looking for structural abnormalities that could lead to problems, including strains, sprains, and stiff joints and ligaments, as a result of accidents and injuries, as well as postural problems or work-related stresses.

- **PSYCHOLOGICAL CAUSES:** Your emotions and state of mind can have a detrimental effect on your physical condition, so the naturopath will want to eliminate negative feelings of anger, resentment, hatred, fear, anxiety, etc.

According to the principles of naturopathy, it is not only the health and well-being of the individual that are important; a healthy population and a healthy environment are also of paramount significance to the well-being of our descendants.

Polarity therapy

Polarity therapy is a holistic system of healing, originally developed by Dr Randolph Stone (see the box on page 92), which blends Eastern and Western concepts of health to promote well-being. The purpose of a polarity treatment is to help the body heal itself and, in order to do this, a polarity therapist will look at the individual holistically – that is, mentally, physically, and emotionally.

The scientific law that energy moves from a positive to a negative pole through a neutral field underpins the philosophy of polarity therapy, as Dr Stone applied this principle to the human structure. The energy that exists in the universe and in the atmosphere around us also manifests itself in our bodies as energy currents, described by Dr Stone as the "Wireless Anatomy of Man".

The body's system of energy fields, which keep the life energy (*prana*) in constant motion, needs to be kept in a state of perfect balance in order for there to be health in the body, mind, and emotions. If there is disruption or stagnation of the energy, this leads to illness.

Who can benefit?

Polarity therapy is not designed to treat specific symptoms, but to encourage healing by rebalancing the flow of energy. Nonetheless, it can be used to benefit many conditions, including:

- Allergies
- ME (myalgic encephalopathy)
- Respiratory disorders
- Cardiovascular problems
- Back pain
- Digestive disorders
- Stress.

Polarity therapy can be used either on its own or in conjunction with other forms of more medicinally orientated therapies, such as herbal medicine or homeopathy.

Polarity therapy addresses many different levels: subtle energy (the "energetic" body as well as the physical body); the nervous, musculoskeletal, cardiovascular, myofascial, respiratory, and digestive systems; as well as the emotional and mental levels. It tackles numerous expressions of disease by unlocking the holding patterns that create the symptoms.

The psycho-physiological key chart (ancient and modern) used for polarity therapy.

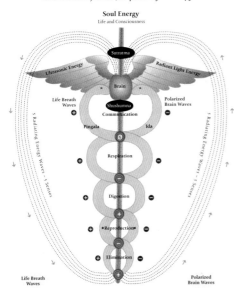

What to expect

During a typical polarity-therapy session of 60–90 minutes you can expect the practitioner to assess your energetic levels using a range of techniques, from observation and palpation (examining by feeling with the fingers) to asking detailed questions. You do not have to remove your clothes, but the session will probably involve both touch and discussion.

During the session your practitioner might incorporate any of the following aspects, which will enable you to take full responsibility for your own well-being – a fundamental principle of polarity therapy:

- **BODYWORK:** The polarity therapist uses a series of "manipulations" or "contacts" via three types of touch – *rajasic* (motion inducing) *satvic* (still holds) and *tamasic* (deep sub-surface contacts) which enable your energy system to seek a state of balance, by helping previously unconscious "tissue memory" to surface. Touch and

HEALER PROFILE

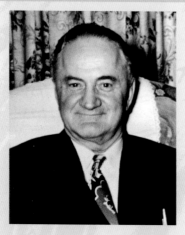

Dr Stone, the founder of polarity therapy, developed a system to encourage the flow of energy around the body using touch, manipulation, and energy work.

Dr Randolph Stone (1890–1981) studied osteopathy, chiropractic, naturopathy, naprapathy (a manipulation therapy for connective-tissue problems), and neuropathy (dysfunction of the nervous system), and gained degrees in all of them. He conducted a thorough investigation of energy in the healing arts over the course of his 60-year medical career. Having published his first work in 1948, by 1954 he had finished seven books of his published findings. In his medical practice in Chicago, he used his new energy approach on patients who presented with a wide range of different conditions, and they reported remarkable results.

He started teaching in the early 1950s and eventually retired in 1973, aged 83. Many of Stone's students continued to research and apply his teachings after he had retired. In 1984 the American Polarity Therapy Association was launched by a core group of advanced practitioners, with the aim of supporting and continuing Stone's work.

manipulation are also used to relieve stagnation and to encourage energy to flow around the body.

• **AWARENESS/COUNSELLING:** Your therapist will allow your inherent "knowing" to emerge in its own time, by building a secure therapeutic relationship. Your increased awareness, together with the release of unconscious tissue memory from the massage, will enable you to realize your own potential.

• **HEALTH-BUILDING AND/ OR CLEANSING DIETS AND NUTRITIONAL ADVICE:** If the practitioner suspects that your energy is blocked or "held", you may well be prescribed individually tailored diets and nutritional advice that will help to detoxify the system. Each person is assessed individually, because no one procedure is correct for everyone. As poor nutrition and digestion may often be a factor in physical problems, detoxifying diets and a health-building dietary regime should be followed, and previous harmful dietary habits should be changed.

• **POLARITY YOGA:** These exercises will help you to maintain your healing process and will make sure that stagnation does not occur. The exercises are designed to retrain and increase body awareness, posture, and balance.

Training

Check on the Internet for the governing body in your own country, for approved training courses. In the US the accrediting body is the American Polarity Therapy Association. In Britain the UK Polarity Therapy Association (UKPTA) is the registering body for polarity practitioners. The International Polarity Education Alliance recognizes the attainment of a specific level of polarity education and offers lifelong recognition of that education.

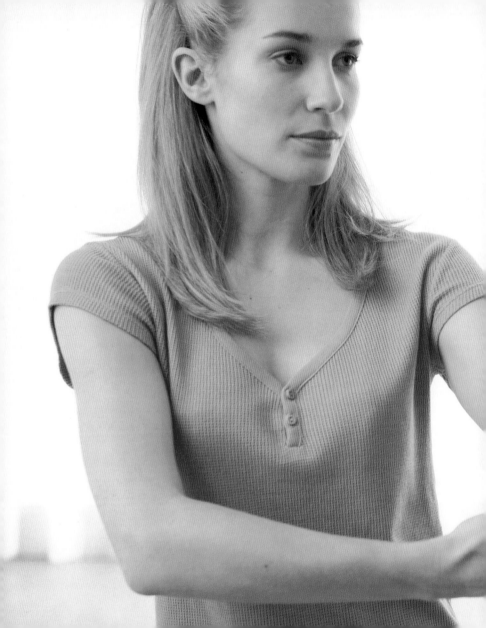

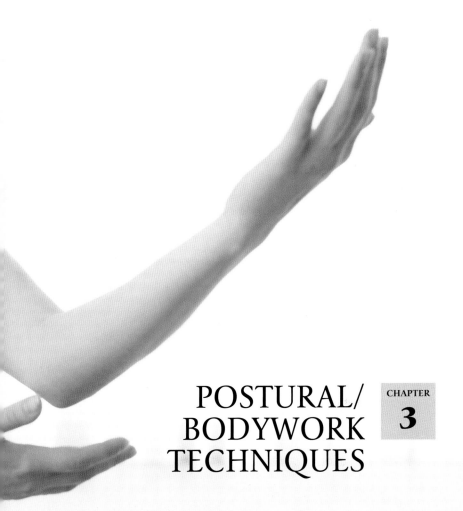

POSTURAL/ BODYWORK TECHNIQUES

Alexander Technique

Strictly speaking, the Alexander Technique is not a therapy, but it definitely deserves to be included in this book. It is about self-healing – an educational method that teaches you to change long-standing bad postural habits, such as slouching or rounded shoulders, that can cause unnecessary tension in all that you do.

The Alexander Technique not only relieves pain and stress, but can also help to improve productivity and performance in any task or activity. It can give you more strength and stamina, and can help you feel more relaxed and think more clearly. Those who learn the Alexander Technique report feeling younger, lighter, taller, calmer, and more confident. It really is an investment in yourself, if you decide to follow its training.

Who can benefit?

Practising the Alexander Technique offers a wide range of health benefits, ranging from reducing stress and anxiety, improving breathing and vocal problems, and lowering blood pressure to correcting poor posture, relieving muscle tension and stiffness, and reducing back, neck, and joint pain. It has even been linked to helping with psychological problems such as depression and insomnia. It is popular with those who work in the fields of music, the performing arts, and sport because it can improve performance and prevent injury. It is suitable for all ages and abilities.

What to expect

A series of sessions with a qualified Alexander Technique teacher will show you how to hold your body correctly and how to breathe more efficiently. Your teacher will guide you through simple movements and everyday activities, such as sitting, standing, walking, or bending, and even

HEALER PROFILE

The Alexander Technique was originally devised in the 1890s by **Frederick Matthias Alexander** (1869–1955), an Australian actor. He was looking to find out why his voice faltered when he was onstage. Eventually, by studying his body in a mirror, he realized that he tensed up when he performed. Over time he gradually adapted the way he held his body, enabling him to project his voice. He went on to develop the idea that the way we use our body – our posture, and how we move – can affect our overall health.

He discovered that coordination and poise rely on the natural balance of the head, neck, and back – what Alexander called "the primary control".

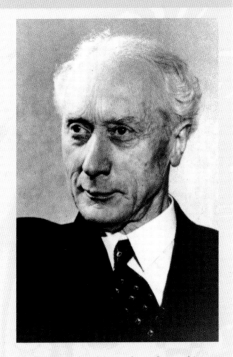

Most of Alexander's life was devoted to teaching others his valuable technique.

The Alexander Technique works by re-establishing this natural balance, to promote easy upright posture and efficient functioning of body and mind.

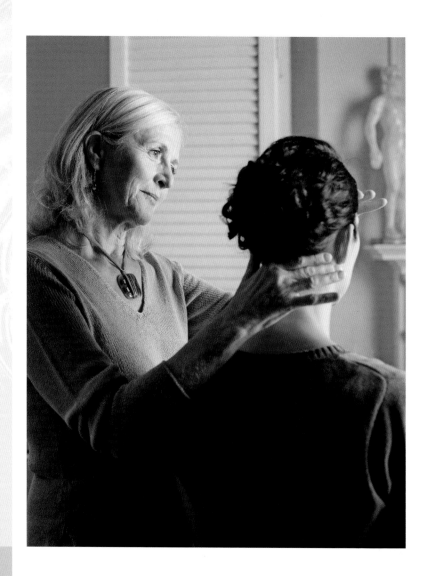

how to lie down comfortably, all the time communicating through skilful hands-on guidance and verbal explanations.

Most importantly, you will learn how to recognize harmful habits and to stop and choose a better response, especially in the face of life's stresses. You will find out how you have been contributing to your problems, how to prevent them, and how to regain control. Gradually you will learn to bring poise and awareness to everything that you do.

It is hoped that eventually you will learn the skill of "use of the self" – namely, how to use your body and mind when moving, resting, breathing, learning, focusing your attention, organizing your awareness, and, perhaps most importantly, choosing how you react in different (and sometimes challenging) situations. In this way you will learn how to swap old habits of movement, tension,

Unconscious, habitual interference with the head–neck–back relationship (the "primary control") affects overall functioning.

and reaction for those that result in a more natural and healthy coordination.

For the best results you should attend a series of lessons – usually around ten – and then have the occasional extra lesson to make sure you haven't slipped back into your old ways.

Training

The Alexander Technique is a practice that is recognized and used around the world, so there is no problem finding practitioners; and it is easy to practise as a teacher at home and abroad. For example, the Society of Teachers of the Alexander Technique (see page 386) has training courses in the UK and overseas. Many of the Alexander Technique societies around the world are affiliated to one another and run their own training courses, so check online to see what is available in your own country.

Once learned, AT teaching skills are fully transferable, so the only real consideration, if you are thinking of working abroad, is the language barrier.

Feldenkrais®

Our bodies are permanently under stress from repeated traumas and bad habits, which can result in stiffness, soreness, discomfort, and a restricted range of movements. However, the good news is that we can re-educate our bodies to forget bad habits and habitual problems, and can relearn how to move with greater freedom, ease, and grace, improving our posture, balance, coordination, and general health.

HEALER PROFILE

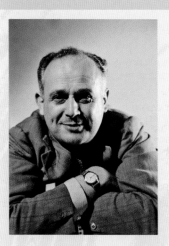

Feldenkrais explored the relationship between bodily movement and ways of thinking, feeling, and learning.

In his youth **Moshe Feldenkrais** (1904–84) sustained an injury to his knee that threatened him with severe disability in middle age. Although he was told that he would not walk properly again without surgery, he decided to use his knowledge of anatomy, physiology, psychology, and engineering – together with his mastery of the martial arts – to heal his own knee.

While he was going through the self-healing process, it dawned on him that you need to work on the body as a whole if you are to achieve lasting effects. These revelations led directly to the formation of the Feldenkrais Method®, which he continued to teach all over the globe until his death in 1984.

The aim of the Feldenkrais Method® is to improve movement and function by putting the emphasis on learning and mobility. The method is named after its originator, Moshe Feldenkrais (see the box opposite), a Russian engineer and physicist who came to England in 1940. He was also an experienced and respected judo teacher.

Feldenkrais® is a simple yet effective way to relearn how to move easily, using body movement as the main means to re-educate the brain. Classes can help you to develop sensory awareness, reduce muscular strain and effort, and regain control over your body. They can also help you to revert to how you were as a small child – that is to say, fearless and physically uninhibited, with a heightened awareness of yourself and your sense of well-being.

Who can benefit?

Feldenkrais® can help all sorts of different conditions, ranging from sports injuries, neck, shoulder, and back pain, and limb problems to relieving tension and muscular pain and increasing mobility and flexibility for those suffering from arthritis, rheumatism, and stroke-related problems. Yet it is not just for the unwell – Feldenkrais® can also benefit those who are fit and well, and can keep them in prime health by offering:

• Easier and fuller breathing
• Greater levels of relaxation and well-being
• Improved performance in sport, dance, music, and drama
• Greater ease in everyday activities
• Increased vitality.

Feldenkrais Method® is popular with actors, dancers, and musicians who want to stay fit and be able to relax and switch off between performances. Anyone can benefit from both group and individual lessons, irrespective of their age and ability.

What to expect

The method is taught in two ways: in a group class called "awareness through movement" and in individual classes called "functional integration". In the group class, the teacher guides students via verbal instructions through a series of slow exercises that are carried out lying on the floor, or sometimes sitting, to minimize strain on the body. The exercises highlight awareness of the breath while moving, and the way in which different parts of your body move in relation to one another. You can begin to play with unaccustomed new movements, as you repeat, investigate, and become more familiar with them.

The "functional integration" one-to-one classes tend to be offered only when someone has specific problems. In these sessions you are guided in a hands-on way through a series of movements, to help you to unlearn ingrained bad habits and unlock a nervous system that is used to doing things in a certain way. During the lesson you will explore how habitual movements can both help you and hold you back from making progress. You and your teacher will explore this theme together. Then, lying fully clothed on a low table, the teacher's hands will gently guide you towards a new way of moving.

Each lesson is unique and is tailored specifically for the particular way you move and hold yourself. With the increased self-awareness that the lessons bring, you will soon discover and implement new ways of moving. As an additional benefit, you may notice that you are thinking and feeling differently, too.

Your teacher will probably also give you recommendations for ways in which you can work on your own, so that the new choices are integrated into your everyday life. In fact, lessons can be highly beneficial when applied to long-term problems, and can help to expand on the understanding and experience gained in "awareness through movement" group classes.

Group classes and one-to-one sessions usually last between 45 and 60 minutes. The cost of group classes is about one-fifth of the price of individual sessions. Make sure you wear loose-fitting clothing for either class, and it's

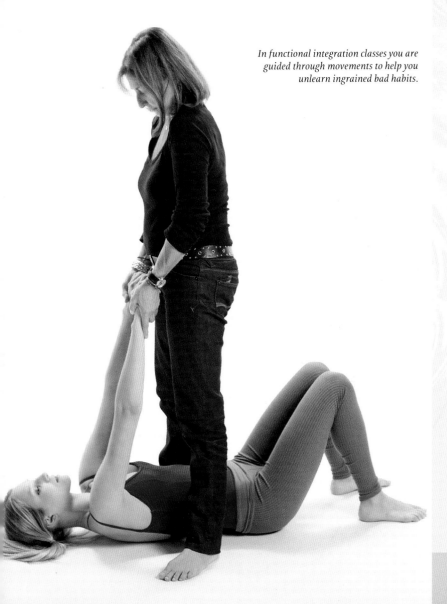

In functional integration classes you are guided through movements to help you unlearn ingrained bad habits.

worth taking a comfortable mat or rug for the "awareness through movement" group classes.

Training

Since the Feldenkrais Method® was first introduced to the UK in the 1980s, it has grown in popularity, with more than 150 trained practitioners now operating in the country. It is also practised in other countries around the world. Feldenkrais® Practitioner Trainings that follow the guidelines set down by the three Training Accreditation Boards (European, North American, and Australian) have established Feldenkrais® Practitioner Training guidelines, and graduates of those courses are entitled to use phrases like the "Feldenkrais Method®", which are controlled by service marks (trademarks for services). The aim of the guidelines is to make sure that there is consistency in the Feldenkrais Method® and to ensure professionalism, as well as breadth and quality in the training process.

If you are training, you should allow time to meet for eight weeks per year, over a four-year period.

At some point during the training you should have an opportunity to learn from international trainers and experienced practitioners.

Exploring new actions teaches you how different parts of the body move in relation to one another.

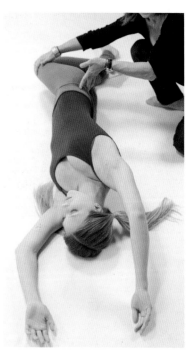

Dance movement therapy

Throughout the ages, society has played with the connection between movement and emotional states, using movement to celebrate, to prepare for battle, and to release anger. But in the 20th century a number of different movements came together to form what we now term "dance movement therapy".

History

The development of psychoanalytic theory at the start of the 20th century, particularly at the hands of Carl Jung and Wilhelm Reich, made the connection between mind and body. The dance theorist Rudolf Laban subsequently developed movement analysis – the theory that close observation of movement would give greater insight into a client's emotional state. Finally, the development of modern dance in the 1920s provided the foundation for expressive movement. For the first time free, creative, and spontaneous movement was permitted and rewarded.

Marian Chace (1896–1970), the unofficial founder of dance movement therapy, began her career as a dancer in the 1920s. She threw herself into teaching, and increasingly found that dance was meeting a far greater need than mere performance.

STUDY FACT

Eurythmy – a method of putting movement to music and speech, which was developed in the Rudolf Steiner schools to encourage and develop children's sense of rhythm – and Gabrielle Roth's 5Rhythms® freestyle dance (see the box overleaf) are both forms of expressive therapy, akin to dance movement therapy, and are designed to encourage self-expression and creativity.

The healing process can begin through simply moving the body in a safe and therapeutic environment.

By the 1940s people had begun to notice her work in hospitals, and the emotional and physical

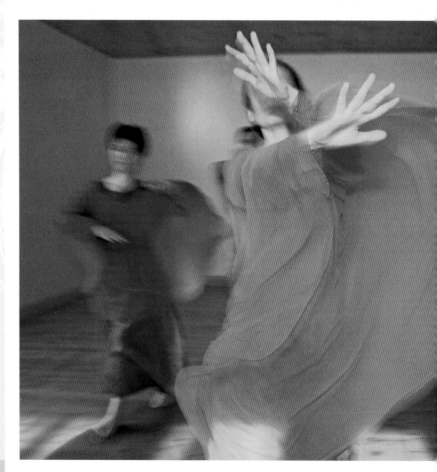

damage inflicted by the Second World War provided a need for creative therapies. In 1966 Chace established the American Dance Therapy Association, and since then dance movement therapy has been increasingly employed in the UK and Australia. It is now found in hospitals, prisons, and schools, but is also an increasingly popular form of self-development.

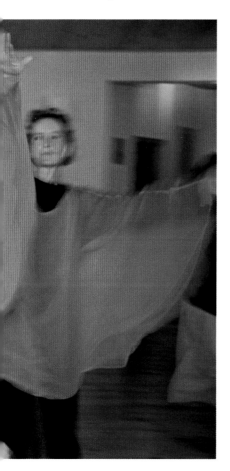

5RHYTHMS®

Gabrielle Roth's 5Rhythms® is a dance-movement practice that she designed to help people explore their creativity and connection. The 5Rhythms® are: Flowing, Staccato, Chaos, Lyrical, and Stillness™, and these are combined with breathing to foster healing and reconnection. Although practice of the 5Rhythms® is usually done in a class, each individual interprets the movements in their own unique way, and the results can be extremely restorative and emotionally powerful.

Who can benefit?

Dance therapy is particularly beneficial for those who find it hard to talk about their feelings, and it is effective for most forms of psychological illness. It is also of great benefit to blind and deaf people, the elderly, those with learning difficulties, depression, autism, or anxiety. It can also be helpful to those with behavioural and eating disorders, or any physical illness that affects mobility. For example, Parkinson's sufferers can benefit from the movement of the energy (*qi*) around the body.

What to expect

The movement of the body reflects the inner landscape of the human being. This is the founding principle of dance movement therapy, which proposes that by moving the body in a safe and therapeutic context, a healing process begins. Both emotional issues and inner conflicts are raised by this process and, once raised, these problems are dealt with on a physical, mental, emotional, and spiritual level. Some dance therapists encourage their clients to use movement therapy to connect to their unconscious mind, and many practitioners subscribe to the belief that by stretching the meridians in the body through dance, you can allow the "energy" to move more freely.

Dance therapy can take place individually or in a group. Sometimes music is used, or a natural rhythm is allowed to develop. The dance is usually improvised, and the degree of teacher intervention varies from class to class. At the end of the movement section of the session, any feelings or thoughts raised can be discussed.

CAUTION

You should check with your doctor if you have high blood pressure or back pain, before undertaking vigorous movement. Make your therapist aware of any medical conditions that you suffer from.

Rolfing

Rolfing is a body therapy named after its founder, Dr Ida Rolf (1896–1979), an American biochemist, who in the 1920s suggested that many health problems are caused by poor posture. In principle, Rolfing is not dissimilar to the Alexander Technique (see page 96), in that it too propounds that improving the body's alignment will enhance well-being. However, Dr Rolf also devised a complex manipulative technique, in order to realign the body's structure so that it can work with, rather than against, gravity. She termed this process "structural reintegration".

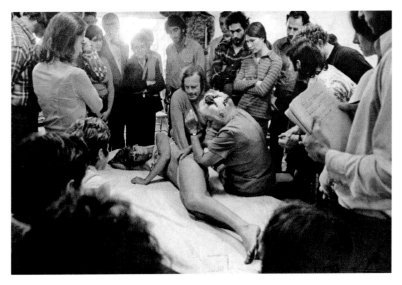

This complex manipulation technique aims to release the stress patterns within the body.

Rolfing is a deep-tissue form of massage, sometimes using the elbows or knuckles, which can occasionally be uncomfortable or even painful, but undoubtedly has great benefits. It stretches the pliable connective tissue and muscles of the body, realigning the system, encouraging energy flow, circulation, and better nervous conduction.

Who can benefit?

Rolfing is not a treatment aimed at a particular ailment, but a system of preventative therapy. Nonetheless, it can offer relief from chronic structural aches and pains that result from poor postural alignment. It can be used on babies and children, although some practitioners recommend only treating children of seven and older.

What to expect

You will need a course of treatments, because each session builds on the last, working on different parts of the body. The treatment starts with areas where the muscles are close to the surface, and then moves on to deep-tissue work in later sessions. The practitioner (known as a Rolfer) may take photographs at the beginning and end of the course, to document the physical changes. The benefits include increased vitality, a better range of movement, and visibly improved balance and ease of posture.

A practitioner usually works through the whole body in around eight to ten sessions, progressively correcting postural problems in various areas of the body. The first session is almost entirely devoted to diagnosis, with the Rolfer assessing your structure,

STUDY FACT

Although people often say that Rolfing can hurt, the pain should be mild and very short-lived, with the relief from chronic pain and discomfort after several sessions making any temporary discomfort well worthwhile.

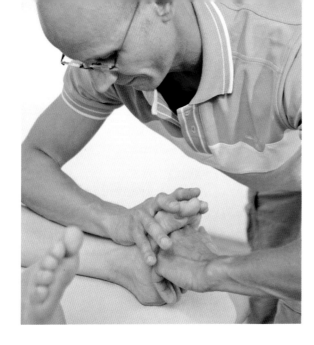

The practitioner's elbows or knuckles are used to stretch muscles and pliable connective tissues.

flexibility, and posture, and possibly taking photographs of how you stand. Looking at the progression of Polaroid "snaps" as the sessions progress is both illuminating and encouraging.

The next two sessions are devoted to the legs, shoulders, ribs, and pelvis, in order to realign the body with the forces of gravity. Next, the Rolfer moves on to the deeper muscles and tissues, moving from the ankles, thighs, and pelvis to the abdomen, back, and neck. The remaining sessions are used to link all of these areas together.

Once you have been through a course of Rolfing treatments, you will often continue to feel the benefits long into the future, as it is as much about re-educating your body and restoring it, so that it can continue to work effectively and at optimum performance, as it is about treatment.

HELLERWORK

Hellerwork is a deep-tissue bodywork programme of manipulation of the muscles and surrounding tissue (myofascia). After training in Rolfing, Joseph Heller developed his therapy in America in the 1970s, as a way to embrace more fully the mind–body connection and the emotional dimensions of this work. By realigning and rebalancing the body, Hellerwork can reduce pain and tension, and it can also teach you how to manage stress, ensuring that you do not store it in your body. It is an educational system and a therapy in equal measure.

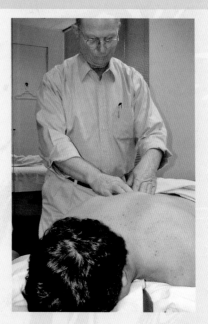

Most people initially come with postural issues and/or backache or neckache, a large minority having had failed surgical interventions. Although on the surface Hellerwork looks like a sort of massage, in fact the work is deeper and has more structural impact, and can be extremely profound. Each session focuses on a different part of the body and the emotional aspect that is linked to it, and the full programme comprises ten hour-long sessions.

According to the principles of Hellerwork, education and bodywork can realign your body and movement, bringing health, energy, flexibility, and self-expression.

Bowen therapy

As an alternative form of massage therapy, Bowen therapy makes use of gentle movements that encourage the body to rely upon its own natural healing capacity.

History

The Bowen technique was originally founded (and named) by Tom Bowen (1916–82), who was born in Brunswick, Australia. Bowen started off treating the injuries, aches, and pains of those he knew locally, and in the 1960s opened his own clinic and developed the therapy.

Who can benefit?

Bowen therapy has been known to treat a wide variety of symptoms, including:

- Muscular and skeletal pains
- Headaches and migraines
- Arthritis
- Hormonal, pregnancy, and fertility issues
- Symptoms relating to multiple sclerosis (MS), Parkinson's, and ME.

It can also play a role in helping to alleviate allergies, and is particularly effective in the summer in the treatment of hay fever: when the immune system comes into contact with a harmful agent, it can overreact and produce antibodies, which release those chemicals that irritate your eyes, nose, and throat. A Bowen-technique massage effectively helps to drain the lymphatic system, which

STUDY FACT

Bowen does not so much "make" the body change, as "ask" it to accept and make the necessary changes.

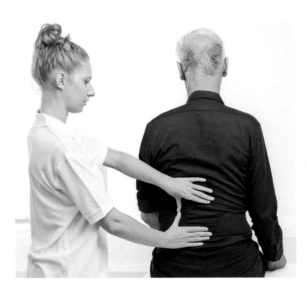

Bowen practitioners use their fingers and thumbs in a distinctive rolling action to both balance and stimulate the body.

CASE-STUDY

One sufferer with acute back pain was unable to move and was confined to her bed, with movement only being possible with the help of her husband, who was caring for her. After receiving Bowen treatment she got immediate pain relief from the first session, with subsequent sessions bringing her back to full functionality.

in turn alleviates the breathing and eye/nose/throat difficulties associated with hay fever. This can then reduce the need for medication and can enable hay-fever sufferers to venture outdoors without suffering from allergy symptoms.

What to expect

The Bowen practitioner uses the fingers and thumbs to make slight, rolling actions over your muscles, soft tissues, ligaments, and tendons, at specific locations

BOWEN FOR CHILDREN AND PETS

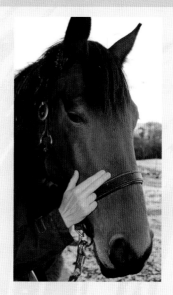

Bowen is the ideal therapy for children of all ages, due to the gentle nature of the technique. Symptoms that have responded well to Bowen therapy include autism, asthma, stress, headaches, and growing pains. The benefits can include better concentration, improved sleep, and a general sense of well-being and happiness. All children under the age of 16 years who are being treated are required to have a parent or guardian with them at all times during therapy.

Tom Bowen even used Bowen therapy on animals, notably horses and dogs. And, following this example, many practitioners today are trained in canine or equine Bowen therapy.

The Bowen technique can be used to good effect on animals as well as humans – especially on horses.

on your body, using pressure that is appropriate for you.

During a therapy session, between each set of moves the body is allowed to rest for a few minutes, to enable it to absorb the new information it has received and to initiate the body's own healing process. Each session lasts between 30 and 60 minutes, with short-term symptoms usually requiring one to three Bowen treatments, and long-term symptoms possibly needing more.

Craniosacral therapy

Although craniosacral therapy (CST) has an osteopathic background – its founder was an American osteopathic physician, William Garner Sutherland (1873–1954), who practised in the early years of the 20th century – it is essentially a therapy that works gently with the body, using light touch and the practitioner's sensitivity.

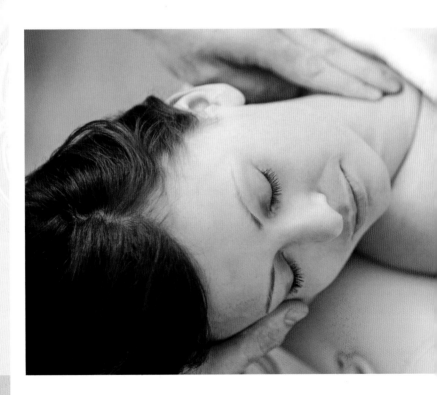

When the practitioner lays his or her hands gently on you, he or she is "listening" to you and your body. Strange though it may seem, many patients report feeling that they have been heard – in much the same way that they might if they had spoken to a counsellor.

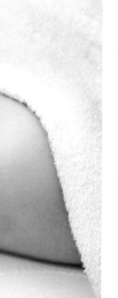

The light touch of the therapist's hands helps her to "read" you and your body.

The gentle touch of the CST practitioner stimulates your body's innate ability to listen to itself and establish what it needs, and then balance, restore, and heal itself. The practitioner senses tensions in the body, and gently helps the body to release them. During and after a session you may well feel calm and yet energized, with greater focus and an increased sense of well-being. CST is great for reducing stress and building energy, and letting go of tension and fear held in the body can help to bring about calmness.

Who can benefit?

People often look for craniosacral therapy to treat acute physical

STUDY FACT

Because the word "cranio" is part of the name of this therapy, people often think it is a treatment that works solely on the head. In fact, craniosacral therapy works with the whole person, and changes can be felt in the body, mind, and spirit, both during and after treatment.

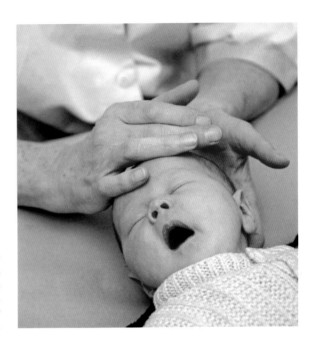

Craniosacral therapy is especially popular for babies and infants who have had difficult or traumatic births.

problems such as headaches or a bad back, and long-standing problems – both physical and emotional. It also has a great reputation for dealing with pains originating in the jaw and recurrent ear and sinus infections, which makes it particularly suitable for children. In fact, because it is so gentle and non-invasive, craniosacral therapy is suitable for anyone, although it is especially popular for children ranging from newborns to teenagers; and, at the opposite end of the spectrum, for the elderly. Mothers and babies often visit a craniosacral therapist for problems associated with difficult or traumatic births.

Whatever your health concerns, beginning to recognize the musculoskeletal impact of external stimuli and internal thought processes – particularly destructive ones, like jaw-clenching – is a useful first step in addressing them. Many people use CST in a symbiotic relationship with the talking therapies (for example, psychotherapy, counselling, and psychodynamic therapy) in particular, and with allopathic medicine.

What to expect

After a written case-history has been taken, the practitioner will invite you to lie down (fully clothed) either face-up or on your side; or occasionally you may be seated. The practitioner will then lightly touch your head, the base of your spine, and then move on to other areas of the body. Don't be surprised if she or he does not focus solely on the areas where your symptoms occur – the body functions as a whole, and the practitioner will go to wherever she or he senses it is needed, encouraging your body to relax and to begin to make the changes it requires.

Although the touch of the therapist is light, the changes can be profound, and some people find this disconcerting. Some people become more aware of symptoms after a session, before they begin to feel relief. Long-standing problems obviously require more sessions in order to treat them, but some people feel better after just one or two sessions. Others may choose to have treatments over an extended period, claiming that this helps to maintain their physical and emotional well-being and that it improves their quality of life.

Training

Check on the Internet for craniosacral associations in your own country and for therapists who are registered with them.

If you wish to train as a CST therapist, most accredited training schools run introductory courses of a week, and then it usually takes one or two years to qualify fully as a craniosacral therapist, after which you can apply for membership of the governing body.

Shiatsu

Shiatsu is a natural healing discipline that springs from the same ancient oriental principles as acupuncture.

Like acupressure, shiatsu (also known as Japanese "finger pressure" therapy) works by manually activating the body's vital flow of *ki* (Japanese for energy) in order to bring about better health. In addition, the shiatsu practitioner uses not only thumbs and fingers, but also elbows, knees, and feet to apply pressure and stretching to the energy lines known as meridians. As the circulation and flow of lymphatic fluid start to move more freely, so toxins and deep-seated tension are released from the muscles, and activity is stimulated in the hormonal system.

After a treatment, most people report feeling calm and more in touch with their body and with themselves. While patients generally experience increased well-being, some report temporary "healing reactions" – in the form of headaches and flu-like symptoms – for a period of about 24 hours. This is as a result of negative emotions and toxins being released. In such cases, if you are concerned, contact your therapist, who will reassure you.

Who can benefit?

Shiatsu is suitable for all conditions, but is commonly used to relieve the following:

- Headaches
- Neck and shoulder pain
- Back pain
- Menstrual difficulties
- Digestive problems
- Stress
- Fatigue
- Depression.

It can even be used for diseases such as cancer, because the Manual

There are a number of different styles and philosophical approaches in modern shiatsu.

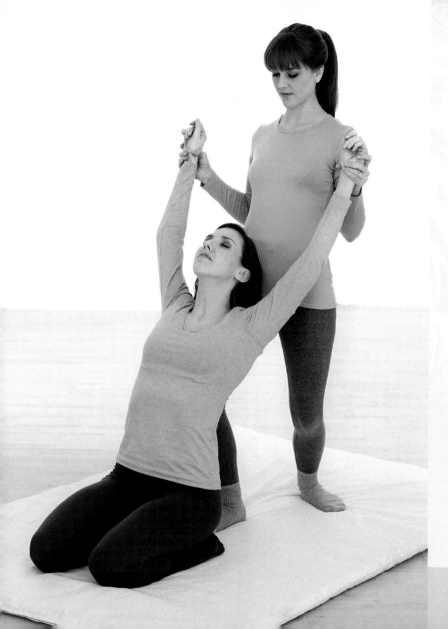

Lymphatic Drainage part of the treatment is not essential and can be left out, given that cancer often occurs in the lymph nodes.

Shiatsu is also beneficial as a way of maintaining health, effectively toning the body's energy; and for relaxation.

What to expect

After the practitioner has taken a full case-history of your complaint and has taken your pulses at both wrists, a diagnosis is made by palpating the abdomen (this is known as the "Hara" diagnosis). The abdomen is seen as a map of the body, which indicates to the practitioner not only your energetic state, but also the relative strength or weakness of your body's major systems. The diagnosis takes about five minutes and tells the therapist which meridians to work on during the session, in order to rebalance the energy flow through your body.

For the treatment itself, you are fully clothed on a padded mat or a futon on the floor, lying prone, supine, or on your side. You may also receive part of your treatment sitting in a chair or on the mat.

The practitioner applies pressure to certain points on your body, using the hands, elbows, knees, and/or feet. The intensity of the pressure varies, and may be combined with gentle manipulations to loosen the

STUDY FACT

Your practitioner can teach you the right pressure points to use so that you can practise shiatsu on yourself as a first-aid treatment, and for the relief of pains and cramps. Many pregnant women learn the shiatsu pressure points so that they can given themselves self-help during the late stages of pregnancy and the early stages of labour.

The intensity of the pressure applied depends on the problem and whether the practitioner is using hands, knees, elbows, or feet.

joints and stretch the meridians, or pathways. The whole session should take about an hour and is usually deeply relaxing, although occasionally a pressure point can feel quite tender.

Shiatsu also incorporates advice on diet, exercise, and lifestyle, encouraging self-understanding and a greater independence in health matters. A personal health assessment may also be given.

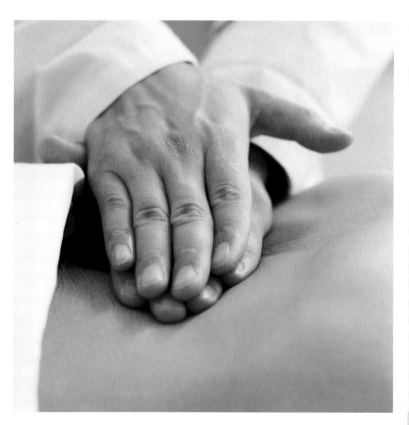

JIN SHIN JYUTSU

Although it is generally accepted that Jin Shin Jyutsu has a lot in common with shiatsu, it is fair to say that it also has its own philosophy and physiology. In Jin Shin Jyutsu the pathways throughout the body through which energy moves are known as "flows", and the different levels at which energy works are called "depths".

Your way of life, an accident, emotional difficulties, or illness can all cause energy to stagnate or become blocked. In this instance the practitioner gently but firmly places his or her hands on the relevant "safety energy locks", in order to release the flow of energy again. Each point relates to a particular organ, joint, or symptom. There are 26 in total and they are located on each side of the body. Holding these energy locks in combination can bring balance to mind, body, and spirit.

You can practise Jin Shin Jyutsu on yourself or you can consult a trained practitioner. Expect a session to last in the region of an hour or so; no massage, muscle manipulation, or drugs will be used during the session. Rather, this gentle treatment relies solely on placing the fingertips (over clothing) on designated safety energy locks, to harmonize and restore the energy flow. This assists in the reduction of tension and stress that accumulate through normal daily living.

Training

Look out for the initials MRSS after a practitioner's name, in the UK – this means that they are registered with the Shiatsu Society, have reached an approved standard of training, and are bound by the code of ethics of the society. All registered practitioners have professional indemnity insurance. Elsewhere, check the Internet for official organizations in your own country.

Qigong

Although qigong is sometimes spelled ch'i kung, the pronunciation of both spellings is the same: namely, "chee" and "gung" (as in "lung"). This powerful system of healing and energy medicine from China uses breathing techniques, gentle exercises and postures, and focused intention or meditation to cleanse and strengthen the body by circulating the vital force or energy (known as *qi*). By practising this system of movements and breathing techniques you can gain better health and vitality and a calmer mind.

This ancient Chinese system of healing even pre-dates yoga, with archaeological evidence suggesting that it is at least 5,000 years old (for instance, Mawang-diu Silk Texts from 168 BCE show a series of exercises which resemble qigong exercises that are still practised today; and the ancient writings of Laozi and Zhuangzi both describe meditative training and physical exercise that are akin to qigong). Like yoga, qigong integrates body and mind to achieve a state of harmony. However, in qigong the energy is moved internally rather than externally.

Qigong exercises all relate to the acupuncture or pressure points that lie along the meridians, or

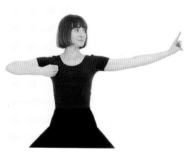

Practising qigong integrates body and mind to achieve a state of harmony.

STUDY FACT

In the past, qigong was known as *nei gong* ("inner work") or *tao yin* ("guiding energy").

energy channels, of the body (see page 18). Different sets of movements concentrate on different body organs and systems, and they can be practised to target specific health problems.

Regular qigong practitioners report feeling more youthful and having greater vitality, and that their health is maintained, even into old age. Yet most advocates of this therapy would say that the greatest benefits are in the form of re-establishing the body–mind–soul connection.

Who can benefit?

Qigong is suitable for all ages, young and old alike, and although it is usually practised while standing, it can also be performed in a sitting or supine position.

The gentle and rhythmic practice of qigong movements

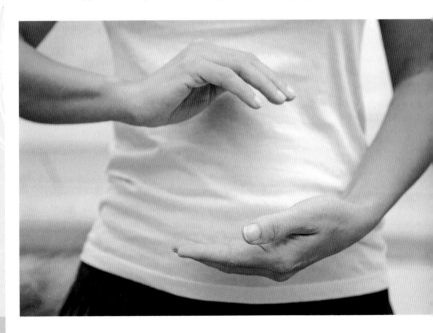

helps to reduce stress, build stamina, increase vitality, and enhance the immune system. It is also known to:

- Lower the resting heart rate, blood pressure, and cholesterol levels
- Improve circulation
- Help lymphatic drainage and digestive functions
- Slow the respiratory rate (benefiting asthma and bronchitis sufferers in particular)
- Significantly improve relief from chronic pain.

What to expect

If you are targeting a specific health problem, qigong can be taught on a one-to-one basis, usually in 90-minute sessions, and exercises are tailored specifically to your problem. Ten sessions are the usual requirement, to get the best results. As well as the breathing exercises, body exercises, and relaxation that you will do

Qigong works with energy. During exercises, you may be encouraged to feel and move the energy between your hands.

with your practitioner, you will be expected to practise at home between sessions.

For those looking for the preventative and self-healing qualities of qigong, group classes practised on a regular basis will probably suffice. You can choose from simple, internal forms of qigong practice to more challenging and intricate external styles. Anyone can benefit, whether you are a fit athlete or lead a sedentary lifestyle, are a child or a senior citizen. And because qigong practice can take place anywhere at any time, you don't have to splash out on purchasing special clothing or health-club membership.

One of the most common forms of qigong practised in the West is Ba Duan Jin, often translated as the "Eight Strands of Brocade". It is the form that I practise at home, and its simplicity belies its efficacy in heightening energy levels and alertness, as well its ability to improve your general sense of well-being and joy in life.

EXTERNAL *QI* HEALING

Often used in conjunction with qigong, in External *Qi* Healing (EQH) the healer taps into a well of healing energy and then "channels" it through to the client. However, unlike other forms of energy healing, EQH includes exercises that increase sensitivity to energy fields, so that the more you practise the exercises and meditation, the more effective your healing treatments become. You will remain fully clothed during an EQH healing. Sometimes practitioners offer gentle hands-on work, together with the energy element, helping to boost your own energy body and to bring about balance and harmony.

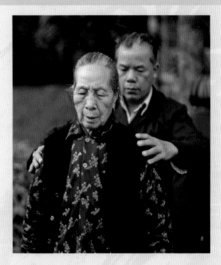

An EQH healer acts as a channel for healing energy, but the practitioner will also teach you exercises and meditation to enhance your sensitivity to the energy fields.

T'ai chi ch'uan

T'ai chi ch'uan is a type of exercise system that has its origins in Taoism (see the box on page 131), one of China's oldest belief systems. Although t'ai chi is perhaps best known as a martial-art form for self-defence, the practice can be hugely beneficial to your health.

In ancient China, t'ai chi evolved to help people stay fit so that they were able to defend themselves against attack from wild animals and bandits; it also helped them with their powers of meditation. Now it is being adopted all over the world as a way to stay fit, improve health, and bring calmness and serenity into busy modern lives. Those who practise it regularly will develop a healthy body and an alert mind. Although t'ai chi ch'uan is the most common form of this ancient exercise, there are variations on the forms that are taught (see the box on page 132).

The t'ai chi ch'uan Hand Form consists of 108 movements (or

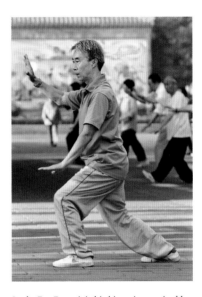

In the Far East, t'ai chi ch'uan is practised by groups in public places and anyone can join in the practice.

Long Form) that are practised in a slow, graceful fashion that somewhat resembles a classic dance. There is no set length of time for practising the Hand Form from the beginning to end, but around 15 minutes is the usual duration.

The aim of t'ai chi ch'uan is to "seek tranquillity in motion".

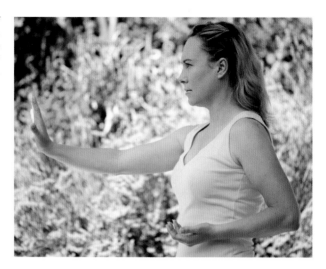

As you concentrate completely on executing these complex manoeuvres, keeping the body and mind in harmony, you learn to regulate your breathing and the contraction and expansion of your diaphragm. This gives the body's muscles and joints a balanced and full workout, and calms the mind at the same time.

The underlying Taoist message of t'ai chi is to "seek tranquillity in motion". This means that the slowness of your movements when practising the forms results in peace of mind, as you lose yourself in concentration on the exercise and forget all other distractions. Let the soft, slow practice take away your tensions and, as a by-product, you may well find that you are better able to concentrate.

Who can benefit?

This system of exercise is suitable for people of all ages and requires little or no special equipment. It can be practised in a relatively small area, either indoors or outdoors, often in group classes (45–60 minutes long), but it may also be practised alone.

WHAT IS TAOISM?

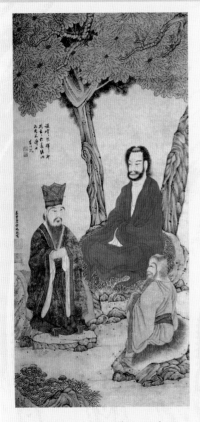

Chinese philosophers, Confucius and Laozi, and Buddhist Arhat depicted on a scroll by Ding Yunpeng (1547–1628).

Taoism (also spelt Daoism, which is the English pronunciation of the Chinese word) is an ancient tradition of philosophy and religious belief that originated in China about 2,000 years ago. It is all about the Tao, which translates as "the Way", meaning roughly the way of the universe. According to Tao principles, all things are unified and connected. This is about Yin and Yang, the principle of seeing the world as being filled with complementary forces: soft and hard, light and dark, hot and cold, and so on. Taoist practices include meditation, feng shui, reading and chanting scriptures, and mediumship.

Taoism promotes:

- Harmony or union with nature
- The pursuit of spiritual immortality
- Being "virtuous" (but not ostentatiously so)
- Self-development.

HEALER PROFILE

T'ai chi master and teacher **Jason Chan** is co-founder of the Light Foundation, which coordinates teacher-training programmes, workshops, and retreats for Infinite Tai Chi™, Infinite Chi Kung™, and the Ling Chi Healing Art™ in the UK, Europe, Thailand, and the US. These unique forms have evolved through Chan's 25 years of teaching t'ai chi both in the UK and Thailand. He is one of the most powerful energy masters I have ever been lucky enough to meet.

The courses incorporate physical-exercise elements with spiritual meditation and contemplation. Chan says, "Through Infinite Tai Chi™ training, the student achieves self-empowerment, self-confidence – beginning to open one's heart and mind." The courses are completed over three years, and many of the students become Ling Chi™ healers.

Ling Chi™ healing concentrates on energy-healing or *chi*-healing, releasing energetic blockages and supporting the nervous system and the vital systems of our physical existence. Chan explains, "It is based on powerful cultivation of the pure *qi* [*chi*] presence by the practitioner. We help individuals to release their emotional blocks through both the work and through the spiritual or light presence from the practitioner. A spiritual presence helps the healing process tremendously, because this is love itself."

Chan says that being in the presence of a Ling Chi™ healer and Infinite Tai Chi™ teacher is the most beneficial way to achieve healing, but it can still be achieved in their absence.

Jason Chan is the founder of the Light Foundation, which offers teacher training programmes in Infinite Tai Chi™, Infinite Chi Kung™ and Ling Chi Healing Art™, all of which were devised by him.

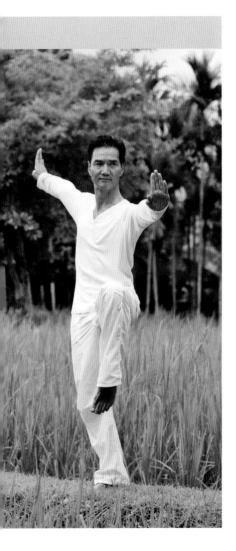

The regular practice of t'ai chi ch'uan can improve your circulation, helping to prevent thrombosis and other ailments of the heart. In addition, it strengthens the central nervous system, stimulates the operation of the intestines, and promotes better digestion; it also helps to prevent sickness.

An additional benefit that is often overlooked is the tranquillity of mind that is the goal of Taoism, and which often results from the graceful movements of t'ai chi ch'uan. It is this that can lead to changes in your disposition, making you more even-tempered and slower to anger. The philosophy of t'ai chi ch'uan is to let thoughts guide your actions, and this principle becomes transferable into your daily life.

Breathing

As we have seen, the origins of t'ai chi ch'uan lie in Taoism, and the Taoists developed a special method of breathing, which is based on the principle of the tortoise's respiratory system:

due to its hard shell, any outward expansion of the tortoise's lungs is limited, so they expand down the length of its body instead, making its breathing deep and full.

Rather than filling your lungs to make your muscles and ribs expand, during t'ai chi ch'uan Hand Forms you concentrate on making the breath slow, deep, and unforced, in the same way that the movements and postures are relaxed, natural, and harmonious; and on drawing the breath down towards the abdomen. This style of breathing is called "the downward extension of breath to the Tan Tin" (a point that lies about 2.5cm/1in below the navel). This rising and falling motion of the diaphragm not only deepens the breath, but also massages the stomach and intestines, increasing blood flow.

Regular practice of t'ai chi chuan can improve circulation and balance and, because it is also gentle, it is particularly suitable for older people.

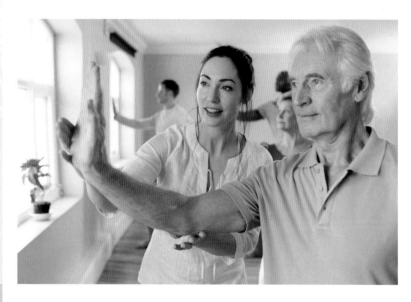

Tui na Chinese massage

Another ancient Chinese treatment, tui na is a form of therapeutic massage and energy healing that, together with acupuncture (see page 18), qigong (see page 125), and Chinese herbal medicine (see page 84), completes the four main branches of Traditional Chinese Medicine (see page 80).

Like all TCM modalities, it is based on the medical principle that disease and pain are symptoms of a blockage or imbalance in the flow of *qi* (*chi*), the body's vital energy. It is the aim of the tui na practitioner to release these blockages, encourage the free flow of *qi* and blood through the body, and restore the balance of Yin and Yang (see page 131).

However, tui na offers much more than just a relaxing massage. Its practitioners are skilled in manipulating the joints and muscles to relieve musculoskeletal pain and stiffness, such as that caused by arthritis and rheumatism. They also direct the flow of *qi* within the body, in order to treat deep-seated problems such as depression and insomnia. Tui na can be used to treat a whole array

of common health conditions and is often combined with the other branches of TCM, to achieve excellent results.

History
Originally called *an mo* (or massage) in ancient times, the term "tui na" was first coined during the Ming Dynasty (1368–1644). The practice is still widely used today in hospitals in China, where it forms part of the front line of healthcare.

In the West, tui na is still a relatively new treatment that is not widely known, despite its popularity in the East.

Who can benefit?
A tui na practitioner will look at the symptoms that you present with, and at the underlying

causes of pain and illness, so it is helpful for a wide range of conditions. Since tui na massage can be relaxing, it is particularly beneficial for relieving anxiety and stress, and for encouraging sleep and relaxation. The

Cupping is used extensively in tui na as it draws the blood towards the skin's surface.

musculoskeletal manipulation is helpful for those suffering from joint and muscle pain.

In addition, tui na can be used preventatively, encouraging the movement of *qi* and blood, and maintaining good health and well-being. This therapy is suitable for people of all ages, ranging from children to the elderly and frail.

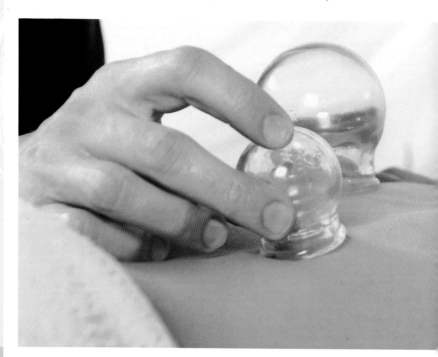

What to expect

After a full medical history, tongue examination, and reading of the pulses on both wrists, a tui na treatment can vary from a deep-tissue, vigorous massage to a subtle energetic treatment not dissimilar to a reiki or craniosacral therapy session. You will remain dressed during the massage and

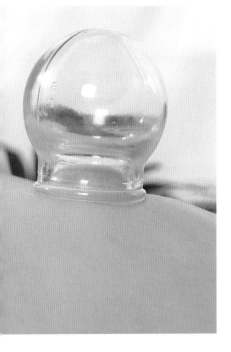

THERAPEUTIC TECHNIQUES

- **CUPPING:** In order to clear stagnant *qi* and stimulate blood flow, glass cups with a vacuum seal are placed on the skin for five to ten minutes, to draw the blood towards the surface of the skin.

- **MOXIBUSTION:** Burnt like incense, moxa (see page 22) is a dried herb that is beneficial for warming and relaxing the muscles, and for opening the energy meridians.

- **GUA SHA:** This involves vigorous rubbing of the skin to increase the blood flow and get rid of sluggish energy (*qi*).

- **HERBAL LINIMENTS:** The practitioner may apply natural lotions, oils, and liniments directly to your skin; these are intended to stimulate the flow of *qi* and improve the effects of the massage, both energetically and from the point of view of eliminating chafing.

STUDY FACT

You are sometimes left with red marks and small bruises on the skin from the cupping and/or gua sha treatments. These are normally superficial and painless, and should soon fade; if they don't, talk to your practitioner about them.

INFANTILE TUI NA

There is a specialized branch of tui na called "infantile tui na" that is used specifically to treat infants from as young as just a few weeks old up to the age of about seven. It is particularly gentle and unthreatening, and differs from adult tui na because the meridian system in babies and infants is not yet fully developed. Check out the Register of Tui Na Chinese Massage for a specialist in your area of the UK, or look on the Internet for specialists in your own country.

may be asked to sit in a chair or lie on a massage couch. The only time you may be asked to remove an item of clothing is if the practitioner needs to use the therapeutic techniques of moxa, gua sha, or cupping, or to apply a herbal liniment (see the box on page 137 for these techniques).

Initially the massage starts off gently, allowing your muscles to relax and the meridians (see page 18) to open. As the session progresses, so the treatment comprises stronger, more rhythmic techniques and point stimulation. The energy work is subtle but deep by this stage, and you may feel deeply relaxed, or even sleepy, at this point in the session. Finally, brisk sweeping techniques are used to remove any stagnant energy that is still lingering after the treatments. You may also experience passive movement of your joints and stretches during this last stage.

Tui na massage starts gently yet the pressure builds and the massage becomes deeper as the session progresses.

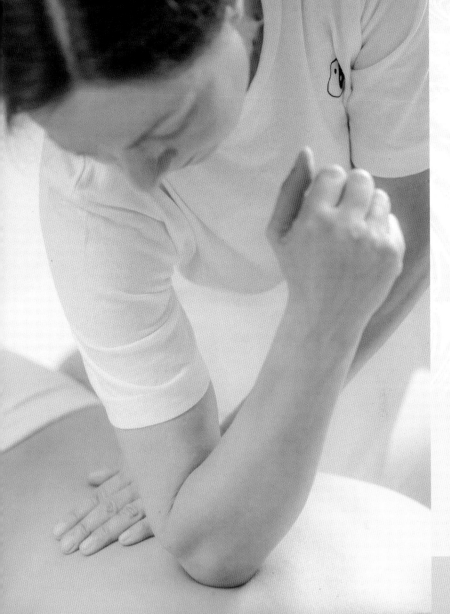

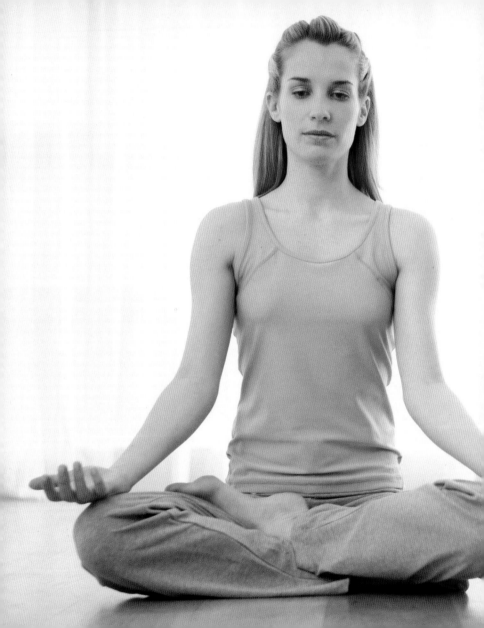

BREATHING TECHNIQUES

Rebirthing breathwork

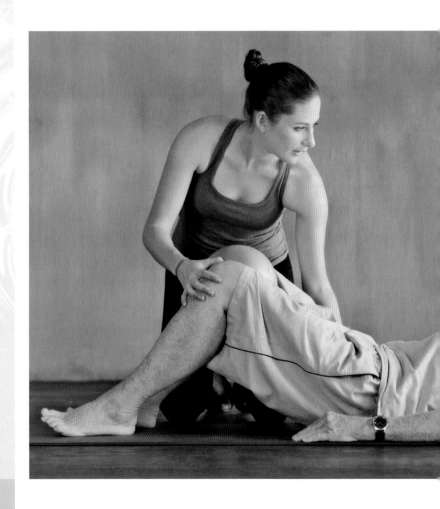

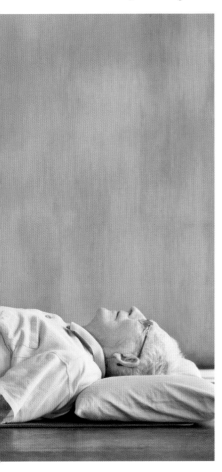

Although various techniques may be used during a session, conscious breathing practice lies at the heart of a rebirthing session.

This is both a breathing therapy and a spiritual practice. Rebirthing-breathwork practitioners may bring a variety of other skills to their practice, including somatic work (relating to the body, as opposed to the mind), psychotherapy, meditation, and other disciplines. However, at the heart of a rebirthing session is a conscious breathing practice.

Rebirthing has its origins in a form of psychotherapy in which the individual "relives" the experience of being born, in order to overcome any trauma or anxiety that stems from the birth. The therapy is based on the premise that the body and mind form a weave of interconnectedness that has a natural tendency to heal itself. It is understood that there is a direct correlation between breathing and well-being, and therefore the emphasis on opening and freeing the breath forms a primary part of each session.

The breath is one of the body's most powerful healing agents.

As well as keeping us alive by distributing nourishment (oxygen) to every cell, breathing is also a main contributor in the vital evacuation of waste material (carbon dioxide and water vapour). What makes the difference between breathing and other healing systems in the body is that we can be directly involved in the process of our own healing when we breathe "consciously".

History

In the 1960s there was an explosion of creative investigations into healing and spiritual experience and possibilities. Both Eastern religions and philosophies and the experience of psychedelic drugs offered new paradigms to existing Western psychoanalytic understanding of human experience and behaviour. Out of this came various forms of breathwork, one of which was rebirthing, which was originated and named by Leonard Orr, who continues to work today.

Since rebirthing began it has spread across the world, being practised by different practitioners and cultures in somewhat different ways, although the principle of conscious breathing has not changed. Each practitioner will bring his or her own individual perspective and experience to their practice.

Who can benefit?

"Both developmental and shock trauma can be addressed with the use of gentle conscious breathing within the holding environment of an experienced rebirther," explains the practitioner Clare Gabriel. "The former includes difficult womb or birth experiences, chronic childhood neglect, or abuse. The latter could involve trauma from experience of war zones, car accident, fire, or the sudden death of a loved one. The discharge of frozen traumatic energy within the body is supported within the conscious breathing environment of a series of rebirthing sessions, and the reframing of the original events is worked through with the practitioner."

Ongoing challenges in our lives can be addressed in the same way. This might include relationship or vocational issues, survival and money problems, self-worth, our sense of autonomy, and more.

The breath also carries a more ethereal substance, known by many different names around the world: *prana* in Sanskrit, *qi* in Chinese culture, *mana* in Hawaii, *pneuma* in ancient Greece. In the West this has become known as the "life force" or "life energy". When you practise rebirthing you become aware of this element of the breath and experience its healing qualities throughout your body.

What to expect

At the outset an initial consultation is offered, at which potential clients can hear what rebirthing is all about and what they might expect to experience. They may be asked to talk a little about their own history and what has brought them to rebirthing. The frequency and number of sessions, and the cost, will be discussed. Sessions vary in length, but are usually from two to two-and-a-half hours, of which the breathing element may be 50–90 minutes.

Generally, at the beginning of each session the client will talk about whatever issues are relevant to them that day. This is an opportunity to be heard, and to reflect in a space of emotional safety, as well as to explore with the practitioner how they are thinking about themselves and their lives.

"As a person breathes in a session, they focus on their breath as best they can, allowing everything else to take care of itself. Emotions, body sensations, thinking all come and go," says Gabriel. "The practitioner gently supports them to stay connected with their breathing, encouraging the natural movement of the breath through the whole system. There are moments when there is a need to talk, or cry, or laugh, or to express what is happening, and time is then taken to explore that with the practitioner, returning to conscious breathing in due course."

As the session progresses, moments of release may be felt in the body; and insights, images, or memories may appear. These experiences often bring added meaning for the client. There is a natural cycle to this way of breathing, and after a while a place of integration and peace arrives, and the breathing becomes full and relaxed. It often feels deeply pleasurable simply to breathe.

Sometimes time is taken at the end of a treatment to talk through the session with the practitioner. It may feel natural at this point to reframe past experiences that have hitherto been difficult to integrate.

Gabriel says, "Rebirthing breathwork reminds us that we are spiritual beings in a material form, and experiencing ourselves this way as we breathe with consciousness is its most profound gift. With practice, we learn to return to the place in ourselves where we know that to be true, giving us a quite different perspective on life. Many people who began rebirthing breathwork as a therapeutic aid go on to incorporate its practice into their lives."

Training

The Global Professional Breathwork Alliance (GPBA) is an international organization that sets standards for breathwork across the world. Many practitioners have joined this alliance, although many others have not and this does not necessarily reflect a lack of efficacy. There are other international breathwork organizations as well (see pages 387–8), including the International Breathwork Foundation (IBF), a global organization that meets once a year at the Global Inspiration Conference (GIC) to share knowledge and celebrate breathwork. Its members include rebirthers and practitioners of other breathwork modalities.

Once the conscious breathing technique is mastered, it can be used to help you to connect with your inner self and to find peace and relaxation.

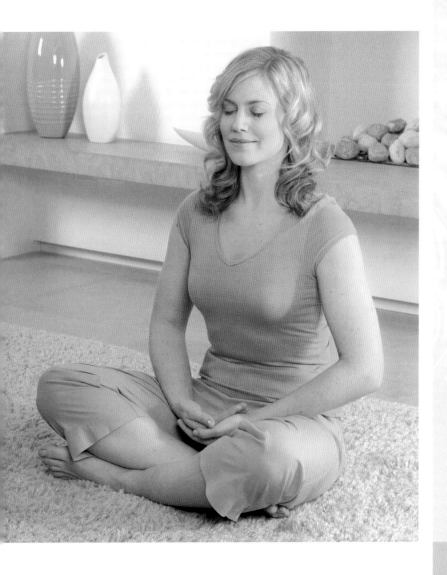

Transformational Breath®

This therapy is a self-healing, self-empowering tool for transformation. It is a conscious breathing technique that works on three levels: physically opening the breath and letting go of physical tension and holding; moving through to a mental/emotional level of release; and opening to spiritual awakening and connection.

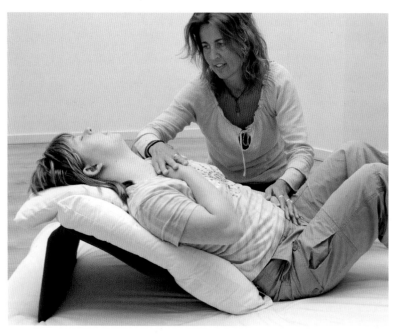

There is no pause between inhalation and exhalation in Transformational Breath®, distinguishing it from other breathwork techniques.

Transformational Breath® differs from other breathwork in that it works with a connected breath – that is, with no pauses between the inhalation and the exhalation. This active meditation focuses on the inhalation: what we receive in life. Transformational Breath® also uses pressure-point bodymapping to support the opening of the breath and the relaxation of the muscles; light-touch acupressure is used to find any tender spots on the body that may correspond to an emotional situation, which the practitioner then helps to release.

Who can benefit?

Transformational Breath® can benefit anybody who wants to transform their life. There is growing awareness that if you change your breath pattern, other aspects of your life can change too.

People with breathing concerns, those with anxiety and mental-health issues, as well as those who need to optimize their breathing to enhance performance (including sports performance and singing) may benefit from exploring Transformational Breath®.

What to expect

According to the practitioner Dr Denise Borland, "A client should expect to be met with unconditional love, to be held without judgement, and supported to deal with their personal goals and aims. They will receive coaching prior to each session to help focus their intention for their session and their life. They will be facilitated in breathing techniques towards the optimization of breath flow. . . and, in turn, life flow."

Transformational Breath® is a "hands-on", fully clothed bodywork. The session will generally take place on a foam

STUDY FACT

Advocators of Transformational Breath® include the founder of the Presence Process, Michael Brown; the author and physician Dr Deepak Chopra; and the actress and film director Goldie Hawn.

mat, and the breath-coach will take personal details from you before analysing your breath, feeding back what they see.

HEALER PROFILE

Dr Judith Kravitz has dedicated more than 30 years to the development of Transformational Breath® as we know it today. With her roots in rebirthing, she has continued to shape and develop this work, and hundreds of thousands of people worldwide have been touched by the benefits of Transformational Breath®. Dr Kravitz has written on this subject in her book *Breathe Deep, Laugh Loudly: The Joy of Transformational Breathing*.

Transformational Breath® is now available in 20 countries around the world and continues to expand. The technique goes on growing and developing as more practitioners bring their energy to the work.

They will then coach and facilitate you to open, connect with, and optimize your breathing.

Training

There are many opportunities for those who wish to learn Transformational Breath® with a view to practising, and several different ways to train. You need to complete levels 1–3 of personal development work, which may be done as in intensive week-long seminar. Level 4 is facilitator training, which includes coaching and hands-on workshop experience. There is also a level 5 training, for those who want to present their work in groups or work towards senior-trainer status.

Dr Borland says, "One of the wonderful things about Transformational Breath® is the fact that the community spreads around the world and there are opportunities to train and work globally. You will be able to work anywhere in the world."

Buteyko

The Buteyko method aims to retrain breathing patterns to ensure the optimal oxygenation of the body and its tissues, and acts as a direct therapy for the treatment of asthma (see the box on page 154). As it retrains breathing, it may also help those who suffer from hyperventilation syndrome or disordered breathing.

Buteyko promotes nasal breathing as a very important part of the technique (alongside reduced breathing and breath-holds). The nose is the air-conditioning system of the lungs: it warms, filters, humidifies, and cleanses the air so that it is less "irritating" to the airways. To promote nasal breathing, Buteyko also involves mouth-taping at night and a nose-breathing walk daily.

Some asthmatics find that Buteyko breathing exercises ease breathlessness and reduce reliance on an inhaler.

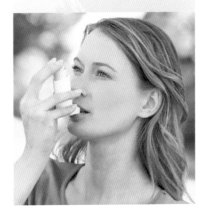

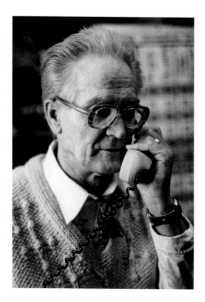

History

The technique was developed by a Russian medical scientist, Dr Konstantin Buteyko (1923–2003), in the 1950s when, as a young intern working in a hospital for terminally ill patients, he observed that an increase in breathing was an indicator of approaching death. He realized that it was possible predict the time of death by monitoring patients' breathing patterns, and that deepening breathing was associated with a very wide range of diseases and chronic conditions.

From studies of hundreds of patients, Buteyko developed the theory that much ill health was the result of the body's defence mechanisms trying to compensate for a lack of carbon dioxide. Observing that patients with hypertension, cardiac problems, allergies, piles, and breathing disorders all breathed more than normal, he decided that deep breathing could be a cause of their ailments, rather than just a symptom. The technique that he developed as a result of his observations is a series of exercises designed to restore breathing patterns to a normal level.

Who can benefit?

Buteyko is most commonly used as a treatment for those who suffer from asthma. The aim is to

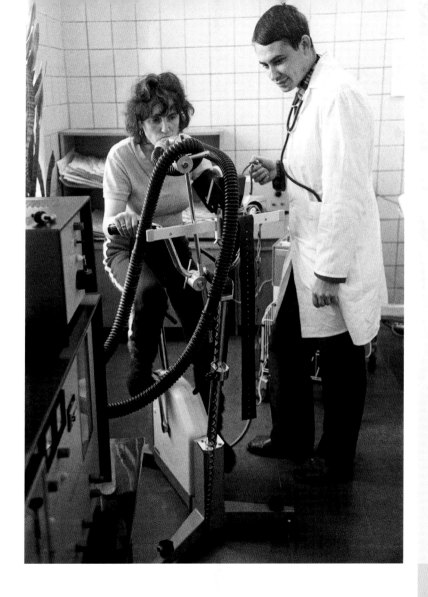

SELF-HELP

A DVD that is available through the Buteyko Breathing Association (see page 388) can show you the Buteyko-method exercises for use at home to help with asthma. A recent study that looked at learning Buteyko from a home video showed that those who used it were able to reduce use of their asthma inhaler by more than 60 per cent in just four weeks.

There are also published studies which show that the Buteyko approach to managing asthma symptoms leads to a reduction in the need for bronchodilator medication, with no reduction in quality of life.

change their breathing pattern to reduce (or eliminate) spasms and enable them to be less dependent on medication. Conditions such as hyperventilation also respond to the reconditioning of the respiratory function through breath-retention exercises.

With eczema, diabetes, hay fever, and other allergies, the treatment aims to reduce the oversensitivity to outside stimuli that is believed to be one of the long-term results of over-breathing. High blood pressure and heart conditions are also said to benefit from practising the Buteyko method, which has had success in helping people to stop snoring as well.

Normalizing breathing stimulates the metabolism, so it can also aid those who want to lose weight.

What to expect

Buteyko is often taught for one hour a week, face-to-face, for five weeks, with patients doing three breathing "sets" a day, mouth-taping at night, and a nose-breathing walk as homework in between. Continuity is important, so you are expected to practise between classes.

You will be taught how breathing relates to physiological function, and the rationale of Buteyko will be explained. You will then learn a number of breath-retention exercises to help establish a new pattern of shallow breathing. This can be quite difficult for asthmatics and those with breathing disorders.

You may also be advised to eat less, and to exclude animal protein temporarily from your diet, because over-consumption of meat and dairy products in particular is thought to increase breathing levels.

Training

There are both national and international Buteyko accrediting associations and they work closely together. Buteyko is often seen as an "additional tool" in the healthcare practitioner's toolbox, rather than as a separate profession in itself. It is compatible with all other therapies, but works particularly well with meditation and yoga. It does not interfere with any other treatment that you may be having for asthma or allergies.

BUTEYKO FOR CHILDREN

Children respond very well and quickly to the Buteyko method because they do not have a lifetime of bad habits to unlearn, and there are some practitioners who specialize in the treatment of children. Nonetheless, they must be old enough to understand what is being taught, so Buteyko is not suitable for infants or babies.

Holotropic Breathwork™

A technique to help you access deeper parts of your consciousness through accelerated deep breathing, while listening to evocative music and under close one-on-one supervision, Holotropic Breathwork™ (HB) was devised in the 1970s in California by psychiatrist Stanislav Grof and his wife, Christina. It is a breathwork technique to help release residual bioenergetic and emotional blocks.

With the eyes closed and while lying on a mat on the floor, each person uses his or her own breathing (supported by the music) to enter a "holotropic" state of consciousness – a term invented by the Grofs to describe the state of consciousness in which our individual

self and our larger self are simultaneously available to us, and material that is important to our further development arises spontaneously. The word "holotropic" derives from the Greek *holos*, meaning "whole", and *tropic*, meaning "movement in the direction of" something (just as "heliotropism" is the motion of plants towards the sun). This activates the natural inner healing process, generating experiences that are unique to each person at that particular time and place.

Although breathers often report having experienced recurring themes, no two Holotropic Breathwork™ sessions are ever the same. And in addition to what is normally thought of as healing, Holotropic Breathwork™ is said

STUDY FACT

Holotropic breathing is faster and deeper than usual; generally no other specific instructions are given before or during the session with regard to the rate, pattern, or nature of breathing.

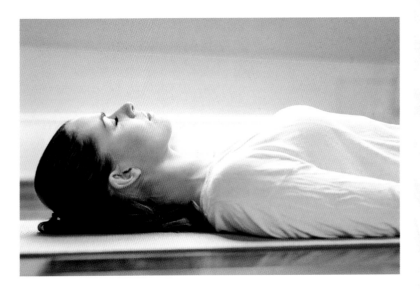

During a Holotropic Breathwork™ session you use the breath to enter a different state of consciousness.

to assist in our realization and integration of who we really are.

It is usually done in a group context. People work in pairs and alternate in the roles of "breather" and "sitter". The sitter's role is simply to be available to assist the breather, by providing blankets, pillows, tissues, and so on, and not to interfere or interrupt the process. The same is true of trained facilitators, who oversee the group and step in to help, when requested; they can provide focused bodywork – or other forms of support – to a breather to help relieve tension or complete the exercise.

After the session, participants give creative expression to what happened by drawing mandalas (circular symbols representing the universe in Hinduism, Buddhism, and other cultures), and are then invited to tell their experiences to the group, if they wish. These techniques help

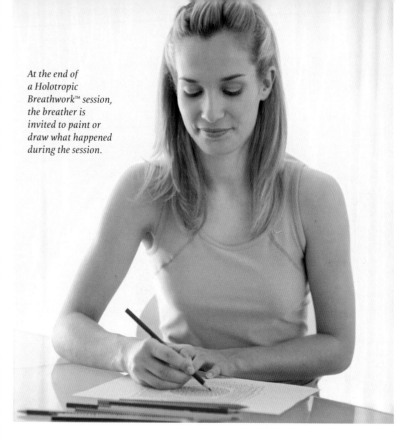

At the end of a Holotropic Breathwork™ session, the breather is invited to paint or draw what happened during the session.

participants to integrate the process. During the sharing and discussion sessions, facilitators do not provide interpretations of the material; they might simply ask the participant for further clarification, such as his or her insights from the session.

Holotropic Breathwork™ can significantly deepen and enhance psychotherapy and other healing and personal growth therapies.

Who can benefit?
The principle of Holotropic Breathwork™ is based on the

assumption that we all have a mechanism that serves as an inner healer, which can be accessed in a suitable context. Your inner wisdom uses this opportunity to work towards physical, mental, emotional, and spiritual healing, and developmental change. Anyone seeking healing for trauma, malaise, illness, or depression may benefit from the practice, as well as those seeking insight or guidance. The Grofs point out that Holotropic Breathwork™ is just one of many methods that can help us experience this healing state, and that all older cultures had techniques to experience it – such as shamanistic practices, chanting, dance, and others – and considered it valuable.

Holotropic Breathwork™ can help you to:

- Release stress or anxiety
- Heal trauma
- Get support through a period of mourning or grieving
- Work through physical illness by exploring emotional issues associated with it

CAUTION

Because of the strong physical and emotional release that is sometimes provoked by a Holotropic Breathwork™ workshop, it is not recommended for people with a history of cardiovascular disease (including angina or heart attack), high blood pressure, glaucoma, retinal detachment, osteoporosis, or significant recent injury or surgery. It is not advised for those with severe mental illness or seizure disorders, or for those using major medications. Pregnant women are advised against taking a Holotropic Breathwork™ workshop.

- Move on from depression
- Access healing and insight
- Expand consciousness
- Tap into creativity
- Experience mystical states
- Access inner wisdom and intuition
- Connect more deeply or get in touch with the spiritual essence.

What to expect

Sessions last for two to three hours. While you are in the role of "sitter", you are available purely to assist the breather, and you then swap roles. Breathers lie down on mats on the floor, while the sitter sits nearby. You should not have a goal or specific agenda when beginning breathwork, but rather trust that whatever happens is the best outcome for healing. The facilitator will lead a guided relaxation to help the breather relax the body, in preparation for the breathing.

The Holotropic Breathwork™ experience is, for the most part, internal and largely non-verbal, without interventions. Although facilitators suggest at the beginning of the session that breathers should increase the pace and depth of the breath, breathers are also encouraged to find their own unique pace and rhythm. Once the session begins, they are not "coached" in any particular way. The facilitators play evocative or rhythmic music as the breathing deepens.

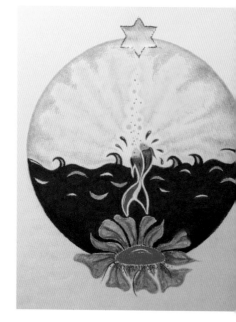

Intricate circular mandalas and realistic drawings of visions are often produced in the final session with the facilitator.

Sitters stay close by, providing a sense of support. The breather can experience a wide range of experiences; some remain very still, while others rock, cry out, or move to the music. Experiences might include deep feelings of joy or serenity, meditative states, a variety of physical sensations, even re-experiencing and releasing past trauma(s) or the birth process. Some people report encounters with mythic or archetypal storylines, past-life experiences, or spiritual/religious awakenings. Many see emotionally charged visual images, feel energy moving through their bodies, receive intuitive insights, and clarify troublesome issues in their lives.

At the end of the session, the facilitator checks in with the breather. If the breathwork has not resolved all of the emotional and physical tensions activated during the session, the facilitator may offer focused work to help release any stuck energy, or suggest that the breather remains on the mat a while longer and simply breathes more deeply and opens up to what arises.

Once the session is complete, the breather is invited to paint or draw what happened during their session within the form of a circular "mandala". This acts as an initial expression of what came up in the breathwork session, in a non-verbal form, and may range from detailed realistic drawings of visions, to completely abstract colours and lines – and everything in between. Often the breather cannot make much sense of the mandala they have spontaneously drawn, but will understand it later.

HOW OFTEN?

For some, one Holotropic Breathwork™ session is life-changing and they need no more. Others use Holotropic Breathwork™ as part of a healing process and attend sessions once or twice a month, or once every two or three months over a period of a few years. Many feel that it gives a boost to their regular form of therapy, so they do a session perhaps once or twice a year, or whenever they feel blocked. Some people choose Holotropic Breathwork™ as part of their spiritual path.

HEALER PROFILE

Dr Stanislav Grof is a psychiatrist with more than 45 years of experience of research in psychotherapy and non-ordinary states of consciousness. With the ban on the use of LSD for research purposes in the late 1960s, the Grofs developed Holotropic Breathwork™ as a powerful drug-free way of accessing non-ordinary states of consciousness. They began facilitating workshops in 1976 and offered their first structured training programmes in 1987. Together they have facilitated Holotropic Breathwork™ sessions for more than 100,000 people from 1987 to 2013.

Dr Grof is one of the founders and chief theoreticians of transpersonal psychology. Grof Transpersonal Training has trained more than 1,000 certified practitioners of Holotropic Breathwork™, who are now offering this method in countries all around the world. Christina Grof died in June 2014, just after completing her book *The Eggshell Landing: Love, Death, and Forgiveness in Hawaii,* a memoir of her own journey to overcome childhood abuse and addiction.

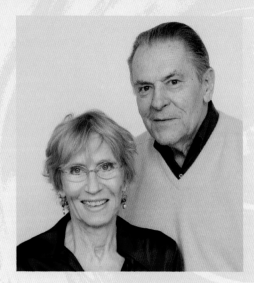

Drs Stanislav and Christina Grof are the founders of Holotropic Breathwork™. Their Grof Transpersonal Training has trained certified practitioners who offer the method all over the world.

Usually later on the same day, breathers and sitters gather in a circle, facilitated by the group leader or leaders. One after the other, breathers are given the chance to show their mandalas (if they have drawn one) and share what they would like to share of their breathwork session. As in a Native American pipe-circle, when one person is sharing, the others do not interrupt or comment, but wait for them to finish, and even then ask before they comment. This is a very important part of owning and integrating the breathwork experience within a safe space.

The experiences in Holotropic Breathwork™ sessions, and what is shared in the sharing circle, are always treated as strictly confidential to the group, and participants are asked not to talk about the experiences of other group members outside it. Participants are free, of course, to talk to other participants about their own experiences.

Training

You can find out about local facilitators, workshops, and events on the Grof Holotropic Breathwork community website, which is maintained by the Stanislav and Christina Grof Foundation (see page 388); it also contains good introductory material for the therapy. If you want to train as an Holotropic Breathwork™ facilitator, certification requires 600 hours of training, which takes at least two years to complete and is offered by Grof Transpersonal Training and other organizations authorized by them. All training modules are six-day residential retreats, and are held in the United States and many other international locations.

Holographic breathing

This breathing technique was "discovered" at the turn of the millennium by Martin Jones, while he was suffering from Lyme disease. Often contracted from a tick bite, the disease attacks the brain and central nervous system, causing pain and overwhelming fatigue. At his lowest point, all Martin could do was lie and follow his breath – which is how he discovered this revolutionary new breathing system, which appeared to counteract the infection. He named his discovery "holographic breathing".

"As soon as I started doing holographic breathing," Martin explains, "I could feel the cranial fluid through the whole central nervous system . . . cleansing the Lyme disease." He also refers to holographic breathing as the "one breath", because the technique accentuates the correspondences in the body and relates to the wholeness of nature as a reflection of ourselves.

Who can benefit?

The practice has been effective for those with dental problems, as it naturally realigns the jaw; and for offering pain relief – including childbirth, where the relationship between the jaw and the pelvis has long been recognized by midwives.

Holographic breathing is also believed to help calm and prevent asthmatic attacks, because it taps into the central nervous system, accessing a new level of consciousness. As Martin points out, "It's easy to be conscious of the body, easy to be conscious of the emotions, but it's not so easy to be conscious of the central nervous system and the workings of it – within humanity, that part of us is often unconscious." In holographic breathing, a higher

Holographic breathing can help you to access a new level of consciousness.

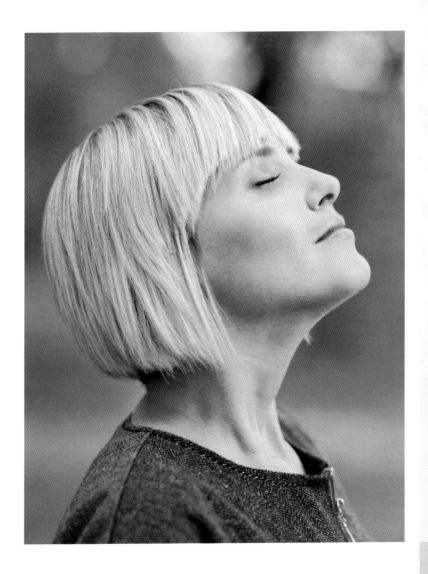

HOW TO BREATHE HOLOGRAPHICALLY

Once mastered, the holographic breath comes completely naturally. As you inhale, allow your jaw to open slightly, keeping your tongue on the roof of your mouth. Keep your lips together. On the exhalation, allow the jaw to close, again keeping your lips together throughout. As you practise, lengthen and deepen your breath and you will feel movements and relaxation spread throughout your torso and around your skull.

The breath is stimulating the flow of cranial fluid and calming the whole central nervous system. Holographic breathing can be done anywhere and everywhere: it is primarily a solitary activity.

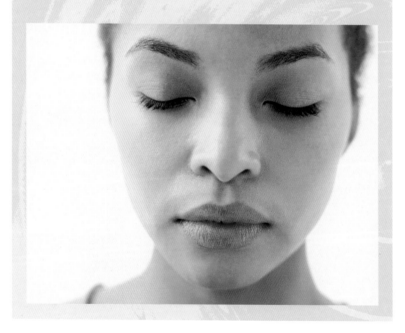

intelligence comes into play to facilitate the meditative state enjoyed by most practitioners.

What to expect

"In holographic breathing, the face and cranium are a reflection of the torso," says Katie McCann, who practises holographic breathing. "The jaw moves, reflecting the expansion of the torso as we inhale. The sinuses are considered the lungs of the face; the outside bone of the maxilla [the upper jaw], the ribcage; the roof of the mouth is the diaphragm; and the jaw is the pelvis. Once the jaw is released, the breath unlocks every cell so that we breathe in an integrated way, connected both within ourselves and with the outside world."

She continues, "In the early 20th century, Frederick Matthias Alexander realized that everyone tends to freeze when they focus on a goal. Moshe Feldenkrais said that we become frozen because we associate success with effort. Holographic breathing gives us a way to thaw: to breathe with and through our nervous system, opening us up to commune with and receive the energies of the Earth and other dimensions. It is a real way of 'letting go'."

Martin Jones noticed that when you are concentrating on doing something, you often set your jaw. However, you can't do that if your jaw is breathing (see the box opposite). As he says, "You have to go about things in a more natural way, you actually have to do it more like water – you have to flow with the situations and the breath to the outcome."

Training

Although Martin Jones runs workshops, the main mode of teaching is aural, through downloads or one-to-one telephone tuition. There are also free tutorials on his website to enable anyone to learn the breathing technique.

Only the jaw moves as you inhale and exhale while breathing holographically.

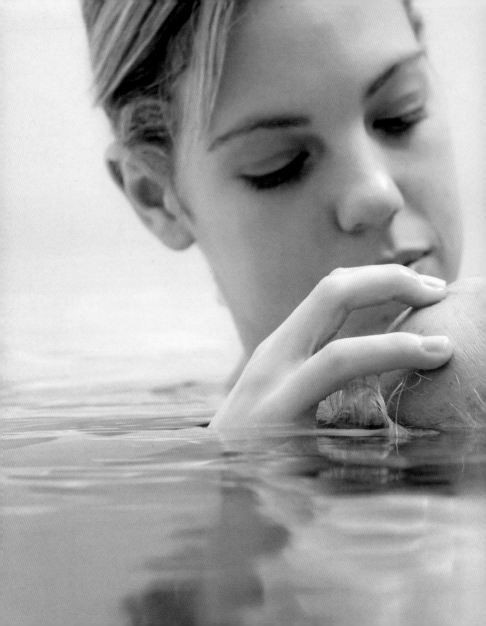

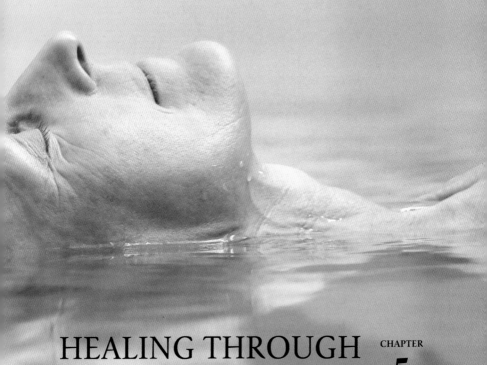

HEALING THROUGH THE SENSES

Art therapy

Art therapy is a psychological and psychotherapeutic treatment that uses art materials and the processes involved as a mode of communication. You do not have to have any artistic talent or ability to benefit from this therapy – the overall aim is to help you to make changes and growth on a personal level through the use of art materials in a safe environment.

Patients are encouraged to express their feelings using the available materials, which might be paint, crayons, pastels, clay, fabric, or even magazine cuttings, to make a collage. Art therapy works on the basis that expressing and releasing confused, disturbed, and threatening emotions is healing.

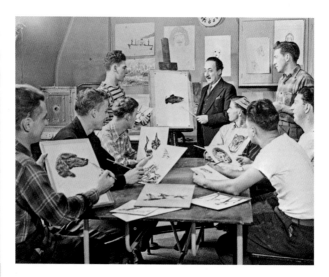

Left In the mid-20th century, groups of artists took their skills to clinics, hospitals, and prisons to help patients.

***Opposite** Expressing and releasing emotions through art can be hugely healing.*

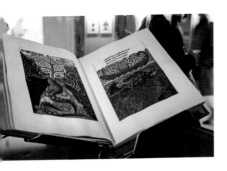

to work in Britain's National Health Service.

Who can benefit?

Art therapy can be particularly helpful to those who find it hard to express their thoughts and feelings verbally. Extensive casework undertaken in North America, the UK, and Europe indicates that art therapy is beneficial for a wide range of emotional and psychological problems, learning difficulties, and alcohol and drug abuse. Recently it has been found effective in the treatment of autism and progressive diseases such as Parkinson's. It is also possible to use it for self-development and creative insight.

What to expect

Before the therapy takes place, the therapist will assess your condition. Expect to be asked about emotional problems and your physical and mental health. The therapy itself is patient-led, and you will not be guided intrusively through the creative process, although the therapist

History

In the early 20th century Sigmund Freud and Carl Jung proposed that visual images reflected the state of a patient's subconscious, and after the Second World War art therapy was used effectively in the rehabilitation of war veterans. Throughout the 1940s, 1950s, and 1960s artists employed their skills in clinics, hospitals, and even prisons on an informal basis. By the 1960s a group of artists recognized the need for a central body to coordinate art therapy, and the British Association of Art Therapists (BAAT) was formed. In the early 1970s the development of post-graduate training in art therapy took place, and by 1982 a diploma in art therapy was recognized as an approved course

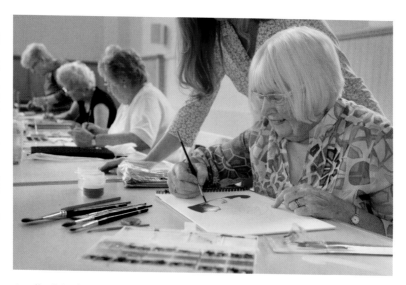

As well as being beneficial in the treatment of emotional and psychological problems, art therapy is also effective for the treatment of progressive diseases such as Parkinson's and Alzheimer's disease.

CAUTION

Make sure your therapist has been trained on one of the accredited courses approved by the BAAT or by the governing body in your own country.
Art therapy can be powerful, so make sure that you feel safe and relaxed with the practitioner.

may respond to whatever you produce with comments and questions, to explore the meanings uncovered and the feelings that have been brought up.

Expect a minimum treatment period of sixth months. Adults generally visit once a week and a session lasts 60–90 minutes. A child's session will last 30 minutes.

Colour therapy

It is well documented that colour influences our mood and emotions and can thus affect our health. First, through our senses, colour has a psychological effect – it can alter the function of brain waves and can lower circulating stress hormones. However, it is now also understood that colour works on an energetic level and can be seen to fit into the expanding field of vibrational medicine (see page 230).

The psychological effect of the colours in our surroundings is striking, and we can actively use colour to stimulate activity or rest, agitation or calm. It doesn't appear to matter where you live or where you come from, for we all understand the psychology

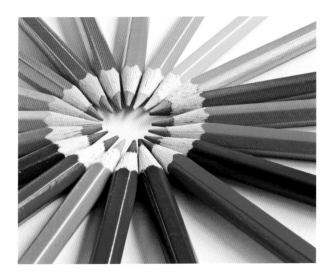

Colour works on an energetic level and can affect the function of brain waves.

of colour, as it is embedded in our biology. If you want to boost energy levels or stimulate activity, red is the colour, because it triggers the sympathetic nervous system. Conversely, blue stimulates the parasympathetic system, which produces feelings of calm by lowering blood pressure. All colours in the spectrum have an effect, as they are recognized by the unconscious mind, irrespective of whether the colour is seen, worn, or applied to the skin. Using colour judiciously, you can thus change bodily responses and restore harmony, and this forms the basis of colour therapy.

STUDY FACT

Many members of the dyslexic population suffer from visual stress, a photosensitive condition that causes perceived distortions in printed text, particularly where there is a high contrast of black print on a white background. The use of precision tinted lenses or coloured plastic overlays can now make reading more comfortable and, in the early 1990s, Professor Arnold Wilkins invented the Intuitive Colorimeter for the UK's Medical Research Council (MRC), which optometrists use to work out which colours of tinted glass will be best able to help individuals improve their reading and prevent migraines.

Who can benefit?

Colour therapy is safe and can be used by anyone, ranging from infants to the elderly. It can even be used on animals. The therapy is often used in conjunction with other natural therapies or alongside orthodox medicine.

In the main, colour therapy is used to help people to bring about relaxation, health, and healing. It is said to benefit those who suffer from:

- Asthma
- Arthritis
- Depression
- Eating disorders
- Circulation problems
- Digestive ailments
- Anxiety and nervous disorders.

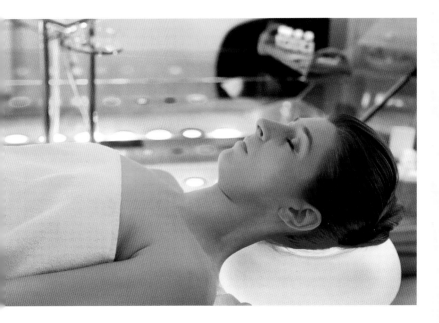

What to expect

After an initial discussion, the colour therapist will diagnose the colour that you need – perhaps by noting which colours you are drawn to, and those you dislike; or by looking at your "aura" (the subtle-energy field that surrounds the human body) to see what colours are present or absent, and by taking a medical history.

Once the colours that you need at this particular time to rebalance

One form of colour therapy involves being bathed in coloured light.

your energy are identified, the treatment will start. This could take the form of being bathed in coloured light (colour is absorbed through the eyes, skin, and the energy field), or it might be delivered via solarized water, light boxes with colour filters, coloured silks, or hands-on healing that uses colour. The therapist will also advise on how colour can be used therapeutically in your everyday life – by eating foods of a certain colour, wearing clothes of a particular hue, and even changing the decor of your home.

Often after a colour-therapy session your therapist will advise getting additional help, perhaps in the form of certain remedies, exercise, colour-breathing, visualization and meditation, colour aromatherapy, crystals and gemstone treatments, nutrition, or art therapy.

Chakras

According to Eastern philosophies, there are seven energy centres (chakras) located along the length of the torso and head. Each chakra is associated with one of the seven "rainbow" colours:

- **RED** for the root chakra
- **ORANGE** for the sacral chakra
- **YELLOW** for the solar-plexus chakra
- **GREEN** for the heart chakra
- **BLUE** for the throat chakra
- **INDIGO** for the third-eye or brow chakra
- **VIOLET** for the crown chakra.

In order for energy to flow seamlessly through the body, the chakras should be in balance,

Colour can be used to bring balance to the body's chakra system.

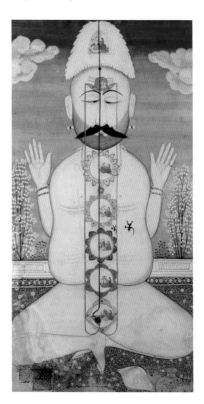

SELF-HELP

Colour can be used in many ways: in the clothes we wear, the food we eat, visualizations, art, and the appreciation of nature in all her beauty.

You can help yourself by carefully choosing the colours that you wear each day: intuitively sensing which quality or energy you need for the day, and choosing your outfit accordingly. Similarly, decorate your house to create the atmosphere that you wish to live in. Embrace the colours in art and all forms of beauty. Include colour in your meditation, breathing exercises, yoga postures, dress, and visualizations.

Colour therapist and author Pamela Blake-Wilson says, "If you need more action, choose red for power, as red holds the creative energy that we all need to manifest anything. For more clarity, concentration, and decision-making choose yellow, but if you become too rigid in thinking, choose the warmer colours to expand the mind; and vice versa if it is hard to concentrate. When more balance and harmony is needed, choose greens; look to the natural world. When insecure, blue is like a mantle of calmness and protection for more compassion; and for understanding, choose pink.

"Become more aware of nature, seasons, the colour of vegetables, the colour and taste of food as you eat and digest and nourish yourself. These are only a few thoughts on how colour can help us. There is much more to discover, within every colour and those in between."

with each chakra wheel spinning smoothly. To achieve this balance, you can use colour. Each chakra is associated not only with a colour, but with an organ/health issue and with certain qualities (see page 276). By focusing on the specific colour and the chakra – especially during yoga practice, for example – you can rebalance the chakra system and restore good health.

Although the workings and potential of colour (which is the small, visible part of the electromagnetic spectrum) are not yet fully understood, it is clear that psychological and physical healing occurs after colour treatment. Undoubtedly if you use colour prudently in your surroundings, it can contribute to wellness.

Some see the body's aura (surrounding energy field) in colours while others see it as white.

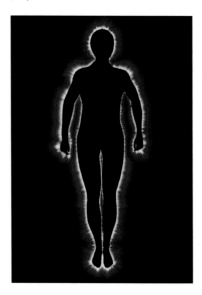

AURA-SOMA®

Launched in 1984, Aura-Soma® is a tool for personal growth and self-development. It is often used by those who want a new personal direction; those who find themselves at a crossroads; or those who simply want to gain more personal or spiritual insight in a gentle way. Using the visual and non-visual energies of colour, it works on the principle that "You are the colours you choose." It also uses the energies of herbs from essential oils and herbal extracts, plus the energies of crystals and gems.

An Aura-Soma® consultation involves looking at a large and a strikingly backlit display of equilibrium bottles (there are 110 in total), containing twin-coloured liquids that are selected to mirror the soul. The top colour is a mixture of natural colour, lotus oil, essential oils, and crystal energies, while the bottom section comprises water containing natural colouring, herbal extracts, crystal energies, and water from the Chalice Well in Glastonbury, Somerset, UK.

You select four equilibrium bottles from the display. Then, using your left hand, you shake the bottle vigorously for a few seconds, until the oil and water combine in an emulsion. This shaking action establishes an energetic link between you and the bottle. The Aura-Soma® therapist is then able to interpret the nature of your soul – and any underlying emotional, behavioural, or spiritual patterns that you may have – from the colours that you have chosen. From these patterns she or he can identify how you relate to the world, and this can be powerfully beneficial for personal growth. Some people choose to apply the liquid from the chosen bottles to the skin via massage, and some put a few drops in their bath; others simply prefer to keep the bottles close by.

In an Aura-Soma® consultation, you will feel drawn to the twin-coloured bottles that you need.

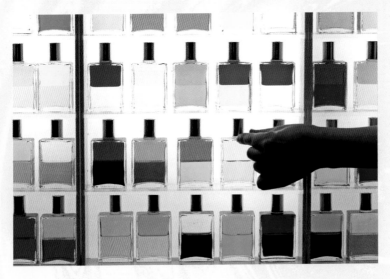

Iridology

Known to many as "the windows of the soul", your eyes can tell those in the know a great deal about you. For centuries the Chinese have used the size, shape, and set of the eyes as a device for discerning health tendencies, while in Ayurvedic medicine eye colour is an indicator of someone's *dosha*, or constitution (see page 74).

In the West, iridology involves the examination and assessment of the iris to determine factors that may be important in the prevention and treatment of disease, as well as in the attainment of optimum health.

Like fingerprints, each person's iris is unique – in fact, the left iris may even differ from the right. Of the five billion inhabitants on earth, not one has identical irides (the plural of iris) to your own. So unique are your irides,

Iris reflex chart

Right eye

Left eye

Right eye labels: Stomach, Brain, Eye, Nose, Ear, Colon, Small Intestine, Shoulder, Pancreas (x4), Lung, Bronchia, Chest, Diaphragm, Arm/Hand, Hip Joint, Ovaries/Testes, Rectum, Pelvis, Leg/Foot, Kidney, Uterus/Penis, Bladder, Teeth, Tonsils, Throat, Bronchia, Thyroid, Trachea, Esophagus, Scapula, Diaphragm, Back, Spine, Liver

Left eye labels: Nose, Eye, Brain, Stomach, Small Intestine, Colon, Ear, Shoulder, Aorta, Lung, Bronchia, Heart, Chest, Diaphragm, Arm/Hand, Spleen, Hip Joint, Ovaries/Testes, Rectum, Pelvis, Leg/Foot, Kidney, Uterus/Penis

as a result of the variations in colour and texture (and, more importantly, the distribution of distinguishable characteristics, such as rings, filaments, freckles, striations, pits, and dark areas), that iris-identification security systems are approximately ten times more secure than fingertip security systems.

Taking a broad perspective, lacklustre or bloodshot eyes are commonly recognized as a sign that someone is feeling below par, whereas a sparkle in the eyes is an indication of good health and happiness. However, to the professional iridologist the 200 or so differentiating signs that can be charted in the average iris can convey a great deal about someone's constitution and current health status.

What to expect

Using an iris reflex chart, iridologists divide the eye into 12 sections, each corresponding

The iris reflex chart shows the iris of both eyes and the areas that correspond to other areas/organs of the body.

to an area/organ of the body (in a similar way to reflexology, see page 64), and examine them using a magnifying glass in order to glean a diagnosis. Iridologists use this diagnosis to warn you of potential health problems, which are usually regarded as a matter of genetic probability – this does not mean that a diagnosis is written in stone, but that there are strong "predispositions" arising from your genetic inheritance. Iridology can help you take preventative action, thereby avoiding what might manifest as future problems. Basically, you can make appropriate lifestyle choices, choose therapies, and so on, if you know there is a strong likelihood of certain conditions being present in your genetic make-up.

Another consideration is eye colour, which influences your physiological behavioural modes. The three basic constitutional iris types consist of the two "pure" colours (namely, blue and brown) and the mixed iris (namely, green or hazel). Eye colour, which is a genetically inherited characteristic, determines your constitutional

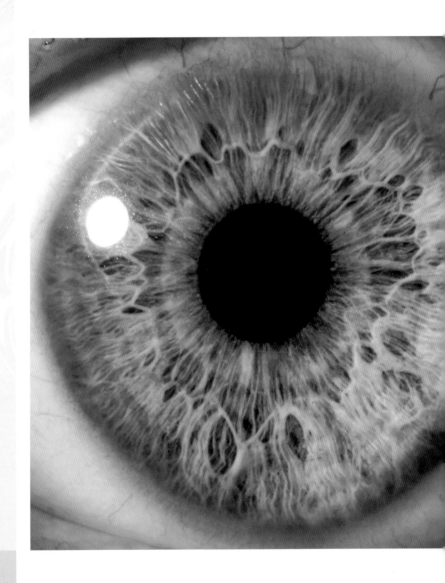

type and its inherent strengths and weaknesses. Peter Jackson-Main's book, *Practical Iridology*, explains to which complaints each constitutional type is prone, and then offers advice on how best to live with your particular constitution, including guidance on diet, health-promoting activity, and exercise.

Another indicator that the iridologist may use to discover your particular strengths, weaknesses, opportunities, and threats (regarding your physical and mental health) is the proportional size of your pupil to your iris. This can indicate whether or not you are an extrovert or introvert type, and the affect this may have on your nervous system.

The next aspect to take into account is the structure of the iris. Again, you will fall into a certain structural category,

THE DOMINANT EYE

A person's right iris relates mainly to their father's genetic contribution, and their left iris to their mother's. Whichever iris has the most outstanding signs is the dominant one – and so if a patient's right iris is dominant, the paternal genes are most influential.

which has a large influence on your constitutional type. *Practical Iridology* outlines the classification system that differentiates between common structural types and their meanings, in terms of physiological function and the energetic behaviour of the body.

Taking all the above factors into account, iridology enables the practitioner to make a health assessment and, from this, to ascertain your particular constitution and how to avoid potential health problems.

Iridology is used purely to make an analysis of the situation and, as

An iridologist uses various indicators in the eyes to determine your constitutional type, and strengths and weaknesses that you may have.

such, just one session is probably required. It is not in itself a therapy. Usually the practitioner practises a therapy alongside iridology – often herbal medicine, homeopathy, naturopathy, or nutritional therapy. There are also a few medical physicians who use iridology.

On every continent, excellent research centres for iridology are now investigating the use of thin beams of light, directed at specific sites in the iris, to stimulate the body's organs that correlate to these sites on the reflex chart. This suggests the possibility that the nerve endings in the iris are somehow transferring energy (in the form of "light") to the organs of the body to which they are reflexologically connected.

STUDY FACTS

Sclerology is another technique for evaluating health through signs that appear in the eyes, but this time it is the whites of the eyes that are studied.

Green eyes are not actually green. The basic colour of the iris is either blue or grey, and over this appears a thin layer of yellow or light-brown pigment, which the observer sees as green.

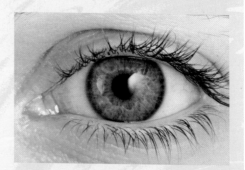

In sclerology, it is the whites of the eyes rather than the irides that are examined.

Bates method

Most vision-improvement systems are based on the work of Dr W H Bates (1860–1931), an ophthalmologist (a medical doctor specializing in problems of the eye) who worked at the New York Eye and Ear Infirmary at the beginning of the 20th century. In the course of his work, examining 30,000 pairs of eyes each year, he noticed a considerable variation in individuals' measured focusing power. This was at odds with the prevailing belief that focusing problems were static and could only be "corrected" with lenses.

He developed a system of exercises for the muscles around the eye and was soon taking away people's glasses, encouraging them to relax, and curing their myopia. He had case-studies published in several medical journals, and by 1911 was working with schools to prevent children from developing myopia in the first place.

In 1920 Dr Bates published the original vision-improvement book, *The Cure of Imperfect Sight by Treatment Without Glasses*, which is also known as *Perfect Sight Without Glasses*.

History

The process of the eye adjusting its focus to bring an object into focus is called "accommodation". By Dr Bates's time it was generally accepted that accommodation was brought about by the "crystalline lens" (a small jelly-like ball inside the eye) changing its shape under the control of a ring of muscle called the "ciliary muscle".

This belief had been established by the English physicist Thomas Young, one hundred years earlier. Young had observed the reflection of a candle flame on the front of the eye. He could see a reflection on the cornea (the clear, curved window at the front of the eye) and another on the front of the crystalline lens. He could see the reflection on the lens change size as the eye accommodated, thus showing that the lens changed shape to focus the eye. Young's work was later verified by Hermann von Helmholtz and others in the 1850s. However, Dr Bates developed his own explanation for Young's observations.

Cataracts (a clouding of the crystalline lens, obscuring vision)

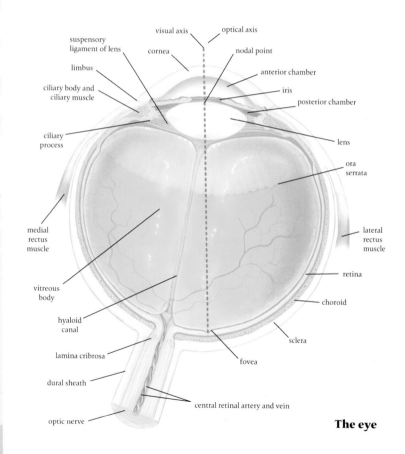

The eye

are treated by the removal of the lens. Some cataract patients, Dr Bates noted, were able to accommodate (bring an object into focus) despite the absence of the crystalline lens. He took this to mean that the lens is not involved in the accommodation process. He came to believe that the eye's external muscles, which direct the gaze, were also changing the length of the eyeball to bring about accommodation. He believed that these muscles were responsible for myopia. Bates's rejection of the accepted model brought about his alienation from the establishment, and the dismissal of his work and methods – and, consequently, of vision improvement in general. This rift remained for almost one hundred years.

Eye basics

The purpose of the eye is to form an image of an external object on the light-sensitive retina at the back of the eye. To do this, light is bent by the curve on the cornea acting as a lens. The light then passes through the pupil, which can adjust for brightness, and is bent a little more by the crystalline lens, to form an image.

The crystalline lens is flexible and is pulled into a flatter shape by fibres pulling outwards around its edge. The fibres are controlled by the ring-shaped ciliary muscle. When the ciliary muscle contracts, it releases tension from the lens, allowing it to fatten, to give extra focusing power for close-focusing. When the ciliary muscle relaxes back against the eyeball, the fibres pull tight, flattening the lens and reducing its focusing power, so as to focus on distant objects. To find out where to focus, the eye first uses information from the convergence of the eyes to find an approximate focus; it then moves its focus back and forth a little to find which way gives a sharper image, and moves in that direction.

An illustration showing the anatomy of the eye. Dr Bates's method uses a series of exercises to retrain the eye muscles.

PINHOLE GLASSES

When the eye is faced with a blurred image, it moves the focus back and forth, "hunting" for the sharpest image. If the image is too blurred, it cannot tell which way to go. If the blur is reduced slightly, by looking through a small hole, the eye can then find a sharper image in one direction, and keeps moving that way until it finds the sharpest image.

This is the principle of "pinhole glasses", which have a screen perforated with many small holes set within a spectacle frame. Looking through the small holes encourages the eyes to focus beyond their habitual range.

For presbyopia (the loss of the eye's ability to focus on close objects as you age), a few minutes of reading each day using the pinhole glasses can exercise and build up the ciliary muscle to overcome the increasing stiffness of the lens, thereby recovering lost accommodation and the ability to focus close up.

For myopia (near-sightedness), using pinhole glasses to focus further away than is normally possible will profoundly relax the circular ciliary muscle and correspondingly tighten the longitudinal fibres. If this technique is practised last thing at night, then the eyes tend to stay in this state overnight, thereby speeding recovery. Not surprisingly, pinhole glasses have become increasingly popular with vision-improvement teachers for use on their clients.

The general principle for working with pinhole glasses is to use them to help you focus in situations where you normally have a problem. If you can't see small print, then use them to read with for 15 minutes a day; within a few weeks the small print will be easy to see again. Conversely, if you can't see things in the distance, use pinhole glasses to watch television or for sitting outside. The most important thing to remember is to relax.

Looking through the small holes of the pinhole glasses encourages the eyes to focus beyond their usual range.

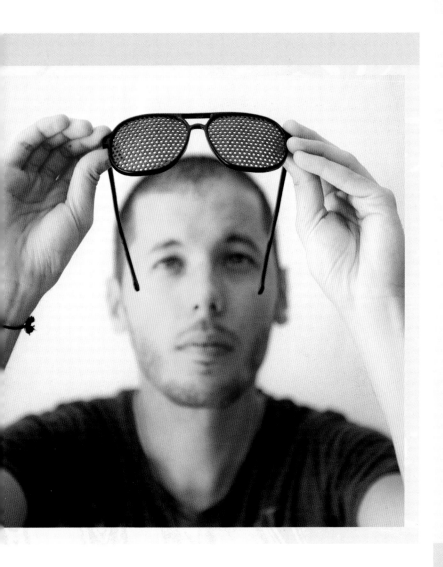

RELAXATION

What all vision-improvement systems for myopia have in common are reduced prescriptions and relaxation. The reduced prescription means that the eye does not have to work so hard to focus close to; the circular fibres of the ciliary muscle are more relaxed and the longitudinal fibres are tighter (see Eye Basics on page 187).

A relaxed attitude to seeing counteracts the tendency to "try" to focus in the distance, which can be counterproductive. The relaxation of the circular fibres can give some immediate improvement to distance vision, while the tightening of the longitudinal fibres brings about long-term shortening of the eyeball and thus reduces myopia.

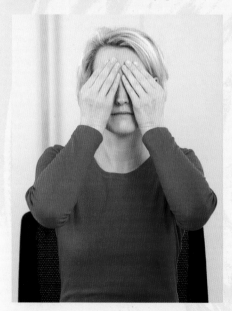

One relaxation exercise for the eyes is "palming", which is used in yoga. This involves covering the eyes with cupped hands to exclude the light. In the dark, the eye reverts to dark focus or "tonic accommodation", which in the normal eye is about 1.5m (5ft) away; this is the natural resting state of the eye.

Palming is a technique used in yoga to help your eyes relax and revert to their normal accommodation.

Therapeutic sound therapy

Like many complementary and alternative-medicine methodologies, the use of sound as a therapeutic tool is thousands of years old. It is now enjoying a renaissance and, with the increasing amount of research and development being done in this area, the reasons why sound can be so effective for helping to improve health and well-being are well on the way to being understood.

There are two main branches of this field: sound therapy and sound healing. Both are based on the use of sound with a therapeutic aim in mind. According to Simon Heather of the College of Sound Healing, "Sound healing is the therapeutic application of sound frequencies to the body/mind of a person with the intention of bringing them into a state of harmony and health."

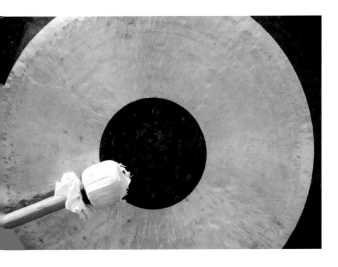

Sound can engender "reflective enquiry" and increase our self-awareness.

Lyz Cooper of the British Academy of Sound Therapy (BAST) describes her method of sound therapy as "carefully considered sounds, instruments, and techniques that affect physiology, neurology, and psychology, along with a method known as 'reflective enquiry', which enables a deep relationship and an increased level of self-awareness to be achieved". This combination, known as the "BAST method", enables a client to gain insight into their personal "wholing" process, and has been shown to be effective in helping to improve health and well-being.

Within sound therapy there are many varying approaches. For example, some therapists use specific frequencies for particular areas of the body, while others allow the sound to find its own point of resonance; some use electronic equipment to produce sounds, while others prefer to use purely "acoustic" instruments.

In traditional chanting and mantras, the vibration of the mystical "ohm" sound is close to the frequency of the Earth as it orbits the Sun.

History

Sound has been used as a powerful and effective tool for helping to improve health and well-being for thousands of years. Many creation stories teach that the world was created with sound. And masters of the ancient schools and medicine people of many cultures all over the world realized the true power of sound to bring about healing and transformation; they were able to harness this power using harmonious sounds, by traditional musical instruments, vocal chants, and mantras (a repeated word or sound, to aid concentration)

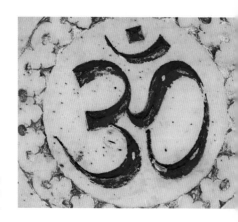

as part of their spiritual practice of restoring the right balance to mind, body, and spirit.

More recently the advancement of new science has provided valuable support and insight to these ancient techniques, and sound therapy is increasingly recognized worldwide.

Who can benefit?

Sound therapy is believed not only to alleviate physical illness, but also to help to balance the emotions and quieten a busy mind. Most people feel calm and relaxed following treatment, and for some people this feeling will last several days. Exercises to practise between treatments may also be given. It is now widely accepted that most illness is stress-related. Therefore treatment methodologies such as sound therapy and sound healing, which promote relaxation and help to reduce stress, can be a very effective ways to prevent and treat illness. A recent study that was conducted by the British Academy of Sound Therapy found that 95 per cent of clients

SOLFEGGIO TUNING

There are some very interesting theories about how certain frequencies are powerfully connected to the human body. Sound therapist Tim Wheater is one of those who is particularly interested in Solfeggio tuning, which he now uses extensively in his music. The Solfeggio frequencies make up the original six-tone musical scale that was used in ancient sacred music. Dr Leonard Horowitz describes the 528Hz frequency as being central to the "mathematical matrix of creation", and it is said to resonate at the heart of everything, helping us to calm the mind and to connect with the Divine.

that were suffering from stress-related disorders felt an increased state of calm and reduced stress following treatment, which enables an individual to relax deeply, achieving an altered state of consciousness that is similar to deep meditation.

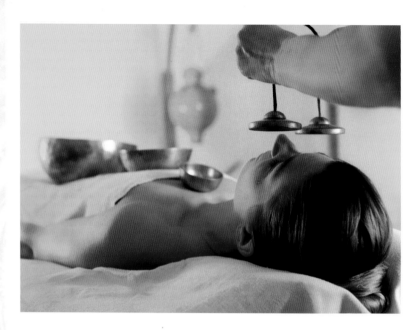

Another preliminary study conducted by BAST measured the effects of sound therapy on the autonomous nervous system (ANS). Clients were connected to a machine (much like a lie detector) that monitored stress responses. Each client demonstrated an overall decrease in arousal of the ANS compared to the control group, who were lying down and relaxing. This study reinforced the findings of other research –

Sound therapists will use all kinds of different instruments during a treatment, including bells, bowls, and gongs.

namely, that sound therapy has a deeply calming effect on stressed-out clients.

Sound therapists have worked with individuals suffering from fertility issues, chronic pain, cancer, stress-related illnesses, IBS, ME, tinnitus, mild depression, anxiety, arthritis, and much more.

Sound therapy can also be used as a preventative measure to help ward off future illness and disease.

What to expect

Before each session the practitioner will ask the client about their medical history and any current health problems, and will then adapt their treatment accordingly, using relaxing or stimulating sounds, depending on the needs of the client. Gongs, drums, bells, bowls, tuning forks, and the human voice are all used.

After the treatment clients may be asked about their experience, and may be taken through a series of gentle questions designed to help them to gain a greater understanding of why they may be experiencing their current symptoms and how they can help boost their well-being. It is not uncommon for clients to experience the release of blockages and marked improvements in their symptoms; others report that the process is ongoing for a number of days.

Training

Training is available all over the world, and courses generally provide a solid foundation based on grounded research and the science that underpins the most up-to-date and effective methodologies. You can follow a tiered system of qualifications, ranging from therapist level, through practitioner grade, to advanced practitioner grade.

STUDY FACT

Modern medicine now uses machines that emit sound frequencies to break up kidney stone and gallstones. This process is very successful at delivering favourable results in approximately one to two hours.

PINEAL TONING

Pineal toning is an esoteric system of 24 vowel-specific tone sequences that tap into deeper levels of consciousness. These ancient and sacred tones, reminiscent of Tibetan chants, are believed to work at a cellular level to aid healing and repair. The vibratory resonances used in pineal toning activate the pineal gland (hence the system's name), trigger your intuition, and stimulate the body's natural ability to heal itself. It is a powerful and ancient technique that is accessible to everyone, regardless of vocal ability.

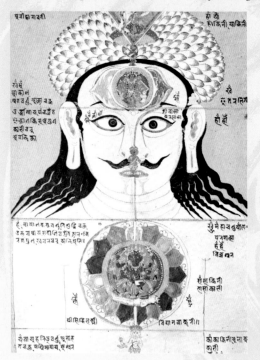

Activation of the pineal gland is believed to be synonymous with the legendary blossoming of the Thousand-Petal Lotus, or spiritual enlightenment – the unfurling of each petal representing a step on the path to greater consciousness.

The Thousand-Petal Lotus is synonymous with the pineal gland which, when stimulated, can trigger your intuition and promote self-healing.

Hydrotherapy

A hydrotherapy treatment uses water to treat a variety of conditions, such as arthritis and rheumatic complaints. A hydrotherapist will recommend special exercises to be done in a warm-water pool (much warmer than the temperature of a normal swimming pool).

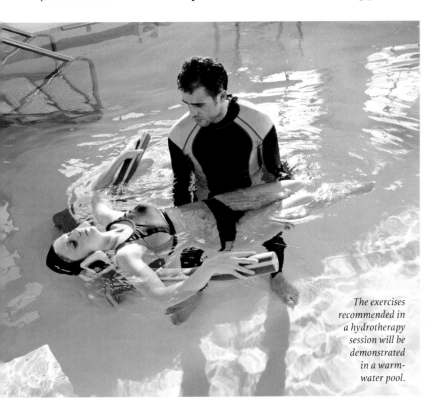

The exercises recommended in a hydrotherapy session will be demonstrated in a warm-water pool.

197

Who can benefit?

Hydrotherapy is often used to help relieve pain. It is a popular therapy for those suffering from arthritis and other joint pain, and muscular aches. Scientific studies show that hydrotherapy can improve strength and general fitness and is one of the safest treatments for arthritis and back pain.

Resistance exercises in the pool can be beneficial to those suffering from arthritis, joint pain, and muscular problems.

What to expect

Hydrotherapy relies on the physical properties of water, such as temperature and pressure, to bring about therapeutic change – for example, stimulating blood circulation and treating the symptoms of some diseases. Present-day hydrotherapy employs water jets, underwater massage, and mineral baths; it can also include the Scotch hose (strong jets of water that alternate hot and cold), the Swiss shower (multiple

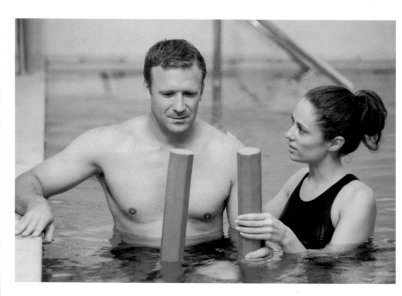

jets of water sprayed from above and the sides), thalassotherapy (the use of seawater), and/or whirlpool baths, hot tubs, jacuzzis, and cold plunge baths. Hydrotherapy tends to differ from aquaerobics, which can be quite strenuous, in that it generally focuses on slow, controlled movements and relaxation.

Most people experience hydrotherapy as outpatients at a hospital's physiotherapy department, where someone with specialist training will explain how to perform the exercises. Each exercise can be tailored specifically for the individual, depending on that person's symptoms.

Before your treatment starts, you will probably be seen by the physiotherapist and questioned about your general health and any specific health issues that you may be experiencing, in order to assess your needs. Armed with this information and with data from your doctor, the physiotherapist will then decide whether hydrotherapy is a good option for you. This initial assessment takes about 30–45 minutes.

Expect the full course of treatment to be up to five or six 30-minute sessions. If your local hospital does not have a hydrotherapy pool, then you may have to travel to an alternative physiotherapy department.

Healing minerals

Many cultures believe that the mineral content of spa water has healing qualities, and so in some European countries hydrotherapy takes place using spa water. Although research seems to support the argument that the mineral content of the water does make a difference, there are other studies that show that hydrotherapy has major benefits, regardless of the type of water that is used. I once experienced hydrotherapy at Évian-les-Bains in France and the therapeutic effects of both the treatments and the Évian spa water were astonishing.

HEALER PROFILE

In the 1990s **Dr Masaru Emoto** (1943–2014), a little-known practitioner of alternative medicine from Japan, took up the quest to understand the mystery of water, which led him to the ground-breaking discovery that water is deeply connected to our individual and collective consciousness. His experiments with frozen water crystals, using high-speed photography, led him to the astonishing revelation that water has the capacity to absorb human feelings and emotions, and to be powerfully impacted by them.

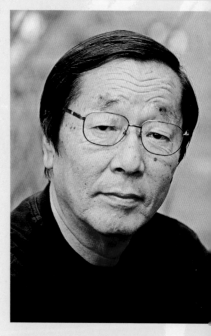

His photographs of water crystals revealed water's receptivity to what he calls *Hado* – namely, sounds, thoughts, words, and pictures. He discovered that water exposed to loving and positive words (such as "I love you", "Thank you", "Angel") or beautiful music (such as Mozart or Beethoven) formed exquisitely shaped and brilliant crystals, while water exposed to negative words and thoughts (such as "You fool", "You make me sick", "Devil") or discordant music (such as heavy metal) showed

Dr Masaru Emoto conducted ground-breaking experiments with water crystals that showed that human emotions and words have a powerful impact on the molecular structure of the water.

fragmented and malformed crystals. Therefore the vibration of good words has a positive effect and the vibration of negative words has the power to destroy.

Humans are 70 per cent water – like the Earth itself – so if we consciously express love and goodwill, we can heal both ourselves and our planet. Emoto believed that since we comprise 70 per cent water, whatever his experiments showed about water could also be applied to humans. He said, "Humans tend to forget things when they get older. In modern science, the reason for this is unknown. What scientists do know is that the amount of water in the body reduces as a human gets older. If you consider that water has 'memory', the reason for this phenomenon (people tend to forget things) can be understood. People forget things more when they get older because there is less water in the brain."

Furthermore, his experiments showed that the most beautiful water crystals are formed when exposed to the words "Love and gratitude", producing a diamond-like brilliance. This discovery has amazing ramifications, revealing the delicacy of the human soul and the impact that love and gratitude can have on the world. Dr Emoto believed that "Love and gratitude" is the fundamental message of water, and the life-giving principle of the universe. He proposed that if humans fill their hearts with love and gratitude, we can restore the beauty of the Earth.

A longtime advocate of peace in relation to water (see the Peace Project box overleaf), Dr Emoto was President Emeritus of the International Water for Life Foundation.

HOW WATER CRYSTALS ARE PHOTOGRAPHED

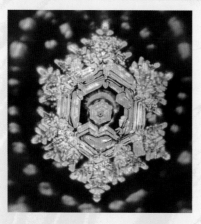

Ice crystals changed shape depending on the nature of the words administered to them.

Water changes rapidly and is unstable. A sample of water is dropped on 100 petri dishes and then placed in a freezer for three hours at a temperature of minus 25–30°C (77–86°F). The resulting crystals are then taken out and put under the microscope to be photographed at 200–500 times magnification. Photographs are taken inside a refrigeration room set at 15°C (59°F), in order to capture the structure and brilliance of the crystals.

PEACE PROJECT

Following the United Nation's declaration of the International Decade for Action "Water for Life" of 2005–2015, which urged citizens of the world to take responsibility for learning all about water, Dr Emoto founded the Emoto Peace Project to help create world peace by educating children about water. As part of this project he wrote a children's book entitled *The Message of Water* to show the need to protect water and to share its message of hope and empowerment. He pledged to distribute copies of this book free to 650 million children around the world. So far the books have been delivered to children in more than 30 countries, translated into many different languages. You can download it free of charge from his website (see page 388).

Light therapy

Light therapy (also known as phototherapy) uses specific wavelengths of light to help treat skin conditions such as psoriasis and eczema, seasonal affective disorder (SAD), and jaundice in babies. But although it can often clear many skin problems completely, it is not usually a permanent cure.

Natural sunlight benefits many inflammatory skin conditions, and it is the ultraviolet light that provides this beneficial effect. In light therapy, machines are used to reproduce ultraviolet light, which is shone onto your whole body (in the case of SAD) or onto the area of your skin that requires treatment (for skin disorders).

Types of light therapy

Ultraviolet light is made up of ultraviolet A (UVA) and ultraviolet B (UVB) wavelengths, both of which are used in light therapy:

- **UVA THERAPY** alone has the effect of tanning the skin, but does not benefit skin inflammation. In order for it to be an effective treatment for skin disease, UVA needs to be given together with a chemical (psoralen), which sensitizes the skin to the light. Combining the two has become known as the intensive treatment PUVA, and it is normally only used if UVB treatment has not worked (see page 93).

- **UVB THERAPY** usually combines both broad-spectrum UVB and narrow-band UVB, but because the reduced spectrum of narrow-band UVB avoids

CAUTION

PUVA is not suitable for use on children or during pregnancy.

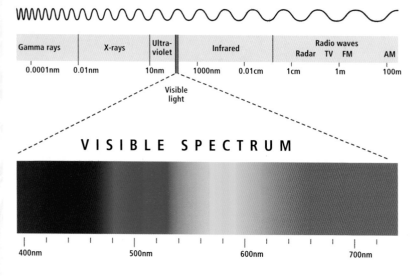

| Gamma rays | X-rays | Ultra-violet | Infrared | Radio waves
Radar TV FM | AM |

0.0001nm   0.01nm   10nm   1000nm   0.01cm   1cm   1m   100m

Visible
light

VISIBLE SPECTRUM

400nm   500nm   600nm   700nm

some of the more harmful wavelengths, using it alone is now becoming the preferred choice. It has the added benefit that it is more intensive than broad-spectrum UVB, so treatment times can be shorter.

Who can benefit?

UVB treatment is suitable for use on adults and children, but children should be capable of standing or sitting still during the treatment. It is also safe during pregnancy.

Above The full spectrum of light wavelengths.

Opposite A phytotherapy nurse will give you the PUVA treatment.

What to expect

You will normally be invited to take a psoralen tablet two hours before you start PUVA treatment. There is also the option of adding a form of psoralen to your bath water – the only catch being that you will have to take your bath in hospital. Psoralen is also available

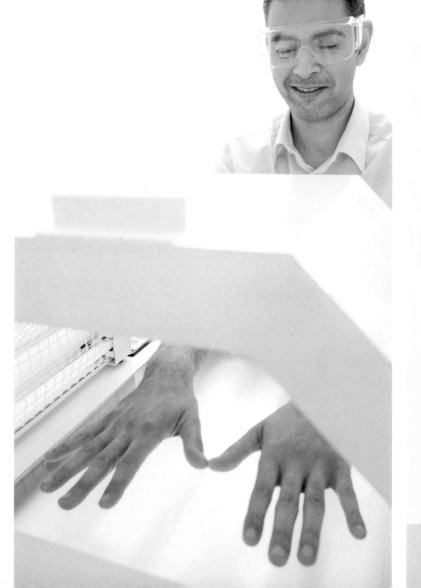

PRECAUTIONS

Make sure that you limit your exposure to sunlight and do not put anything on your skin that might enhance the effects of light while you are receiving a course of light therapy. Your physician may advise you:

- To cover your skin when out in sunlight, and not to use sunbeds

- Not to eat too many foods that contain natural psoralen (these include celery, carrots, figs, citrus fruit, parsnips, and parsley), which can make you more sensitive than usual to ultraviolet light

- Not to use perfumed products, creams, ointments, and lotions, unless you are told to by hospital staff

- Not to cut your hair during a course of treatment, as it may expose skin that was previously covered by hair.

as a cream or gel for treating small areas of skin.

You will probably have to attend your local hospital, where a trained phototherapy nurse will give you the treatment, after a dermatologist has worked out the correct dosage according to your skin type and how prone you are to burning in sunlight. In order to assess the starting dose, a test dose of ultraviolet light may be given to a small area of your skin.

After stripping down to your underpants, you will be given goggles to wear, to protect your eyes during treatment. You may be offered sunscreen to apply to certain parts of your skin, including your neck, lips, and nipples. Fluorescent tubes placed in specially designed cabinets produce the ultraviolet light, and initially you will only be exposed for less than a minute. As treatment progresses, the duration may be increased to a couple of minutes, depending on how you respond.

After a PUVA treatment it is advisable to wear UV-protective sunglasses for 24 hours after you

CAUTIONS

The risk of skin cancer and premature skin-ageing can increase after long-term use of repeated sessions of UVB and PUVA, in the same way that it would from long-term exposure to sunlight. The more sessions you have, the greater the risk, so your dermatologist should ensure that you receive the minimum number of UVB or PUVA light-therapy sessions needed to provide a beneficial effect.

Wearing eye protection will reduce the risk of damage to your eyes from PUVA.

Don't forget to tell hospital staff about any new medicines that you have started taking – even herbal medicines – as they can make your skin more sensitive to light.

If you are using psoralen, you may experience some nausea.

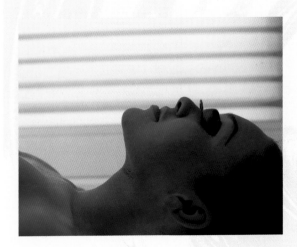

You will wear goggles to protect your eyes during a PUVA treatment.

SEASONAL AFFECTIVE DISORDER

For some people with SAD, light therapy can considerably improve their mood. It involves sitting in front of (or beneath) a light box, usually in their own home. Light boxes contain lamps that produce a very bright light; they are available in a range of styles, including as desk lamps and wall-mounted fixtures.

The effectiveness of light boxes varies and so, before choosing one to treat SAD, make sure that it is medically proven to treat the condition and is produced by a fully certified manufacturer, whose information and instructions you have checked. The Seasonal Affective Disorder Association (see page 388) can provide a list of recommended manufacturers.

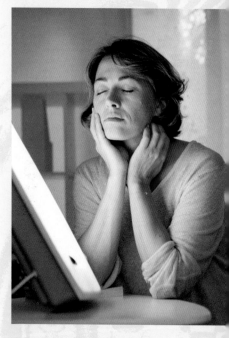

Special lamps that produce bright light can help to combat SAD.

By simulating sunlight during the winter months, it is thought that light therapy increases the production of serotonin (a mood-enhancing hormone) and decreases the production of melatonin (a sleep-inducing hormone), thereby combating the effects of SAD. However, this only holds true if SAD is caused by a lack of light, which is the current received wisdom on this condition.

took psoralen (because psoralen increases light-sensitivity in the eyes and skin), and to cover up your skin when you are outdoors or near a window.

You should expect to attend hospital for light-therapy treatment two or three times a week, and for a full course to be between 15 and 30 treatments. Although in some countries it is possible to have certain types of light therapy at home, there are concerns over safety. Where home phototherapy is an option, you usually start your treatment at hospital and then continue to use a light unit at home. However, it is imperative that you follow your dermatologist's instructions closely and attend regular check-ups. Ask your dermatologist for more information.

STUDY FACTS

High-street sunbeds are not an effective treatment for skin disorders, because they produce a combination of predominantly UVA and some UVB light, which is not effective without psoralen (PUVA) for treating skin disorders.

Prior to the 1960s, babies born prematurely were at risk from a life-threatening condition called jaundice. However, in 1958 R J Cremer wrote a paper in which he stated that rather than curing the disease with a blood transfusion (as was the practice at the time), all that was needed was exposure to light, since full-spectrum or blue light breaks down excessive bilirubin. A yellow pigment found in blood and stools, bilirubin is processed in the liver and then excreted into the bile duct and stored in the gall bladder, from where it is released into the small intestine as bile, to help digest fats.

New-generation flower essences

Although people have used flower remedies since ancient times to promote emotional and spiritual healing, it is only in recent years that a new generation of flower-essence practitioners has revived this healing therapy and brought powerful high-vibration flower essences to the fore.

STUDY FACT

Recently a German flower-essence researcher and producer, Andreas Korte, has pioneered his own ecological method of encapsulating the flowers' energy in water. He has also discovered some unique orchids in the Amazon jungle.

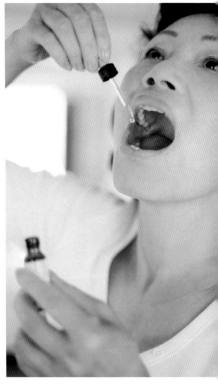

Flower essences are commonly taken by dropping a couple of drops of the tincture under the tongue.

HEALER PROFILE

Clare G Harvey is a world expert on flower remedies, whom I have met and interviewed many times. She is a third-generation healer who learned her skills from her grandmother, who was herself taught flower remedies by the British physician and homeopath Dr Edward Bach (see the box on page 213), after whom Bach Flower Remedies are named.

Clare has been a flower-essences consultant for 25 years, formerly at London's Hale Clinic and the Centre for Complementary and Integrated Medicine, and now at her own flower-essence clinic in London's Harley Street. She runs the IFVM Flower School, with professional diploma courses in flower remedies; has a distribution business, called Flowersense, that supplies major health-food chains with remedies; and has just launched her own educational website (see page 389).

Clare says, "I am passionate about flowers. You can use them with anything: with homeopathy, or if you are taking medication. They are so versatile and user-friendly. The body takes what it needs, and doesn't take what it doesn't need . . . I think of myself as a vehicle to bring flower essences to the people on the street."

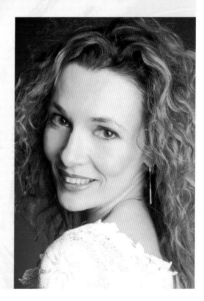

Clare Harvey is a third-generation healer and leading expert on flower essences.

Unlike essential oils, homeopathic medicines, and herbal tinctures, which use the physical part of a flower or a plant, flower essences contain only the "energetic patterning" or imprint of the flower. This positive, life-giving energy works on, and interacts with, our own subtle-energy body.

When our energy is blocked, stressed, or disturbed, flower essences can offer us "vibrational reprogramming", if you like, at a cellular level to re-establish harmony. Each flower transmits its own unique energy pattern or essence. When the appropriate essence is employed, this acts as a catalyst to return our energy to its original state of harmony by restoring its natural frequency.

A flower (or combination of flowers) will be used by a flower-remedy practitioner to match whatever imbalance you may be experiencing. Flower remedies also have a particular resonance with chakras and the aura (see page 176), and in addition they can be used to affect the physical body.

SELF-HELP

Flower essences really lend themselves to self-prescribing. If you are instinctively drawn to a particular essence, then it is resonating with your situation and is right for you. Flower essences work on the homeopathic principle that less is more – so gentle, continuous treatment is the most effective for lifting your mood, creating a boost in vitality, and a shift in energy. However, to treat deep-seated trauma or ongoing chronic issues, you are best advised to consult a flower-essences expert.

Who can benefit?

Flower essences are primarily used to work on emotional, mental, and spiritual problems, but they can also work on physical problems that arise as a result of a weakened immune and/or endocrine system, such as allergies, hay fever, skin complaints, hormonal imbalances, and electromagnetic pollution.

HEALER PROFILE

Dr Edward Bach (1886–1936) was a doctor, bacteriologist, and pathologist who, in 1917, was diagnosed with a brain tumour and given just three months to live. He returned to his research with a renewed sense of purpose, which he believed saved his life, because the three-month deadline came and went.

Until this point he had been researching vaccines, but he now wanted purer remedies that did not rely on the products of disease (the traditional source of vaccine at the time). He began collecting and researching flowers and started to realize their great potential. By 1930 he had left his medical practice and continued to explore the possibility of a new system of medicine sourced from nature.

Over years of trial and error, often using himself as the "guinea pig", he discovered flower and plant remedies aimed at alleviating a particular mental state of emotion. In 1935 he announced that his search for remedies was complete – the result was the range of Bach Flower Remedies that we still use today. One year later Dr Bach died, on 27 November 1936, aged 50.

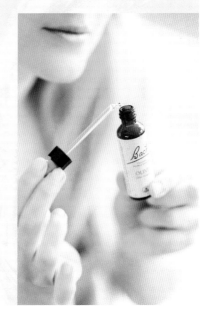

Rescue Remedy is one of the most popular of the Bach remedies and can be used for any emotional or physical trauma.

Flower essences are excellent for clearing shock and stress, grief, relationship problems, and ingrained habit patterns. As the flower essences help you to release blockages that may have been preventing you from reaching your true potential, they simultaneously empower you to respond better to (and benefit more from) the challenges of modern living.

When using flower essences to treat babies and children, you can gently rub the essence onto the skin on the pulse points: on the inner sides of the wrists, the forehead, or the soles of the feet.

What to expect

When you consult a flower-remedy practitioner, he or she will determine the compatible essence (or combination of essences)

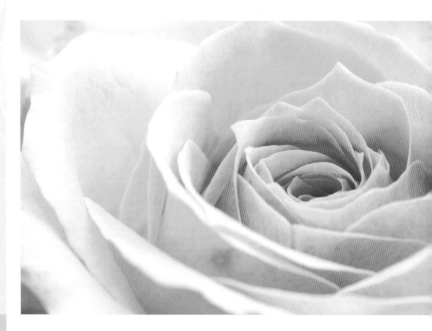

HEALER PROFILE

Dr Natalia Schotte, an acclaimed intuitive healer in the world of spiritual growth, is also a spiritual counsellor. Years ago she bought an acre of land in Michigan and, with a group of like-minded women, worked on the land until they felt it was ready to plant with flowers, which they went on to make into essences. Once made, the essences are held in a sacred space for at least a year before being distributed. The company that markets them, La Vie de la Rose, claims to offer the first and only nature-based system dedicated to "accelerated spiritual growth", known as the Ascension Oracle Solutions.

The 30-essence box is a delight to work with and the flower essences are uncannily appropriate. The dosage is surprising – often the requirement can be for as little as one drop. They can be used in association with dowsing (as I myself use them; see page 254) or kinesiology (muscle-testing, see page 232). The essences also come with a pack of cards – the Ascension Oracle – and you can simply draw a card and use your intuition, supported by the names of the flower essences and their purpose statements, which are given in a brochure in the box.

by using the classic interview technique that Dr Bach preferred.

There are many ways to take flower essences. You can take them as drops under the tongue, or mixed with a little water and sipped – usually in the morning and evening. Or you can use them externally in creams or oils, or add drops of flower essence to the bath. You can also absorb them, by spraying them as spritz into the air or onto your aura.

Rose is just one of the many flowers that can be used as an individual essence.

Music therapy

Music therapy can help people whose lives have been adversely affected by illness, injury, or disability. Music plays an important role in everyday life: it can be stimulating or relaxing, cheerful or melancholy, and it can effortlessly take you back to a different time or event, or resonate strongly with your feelings, so that you can express them and communicate them to others.

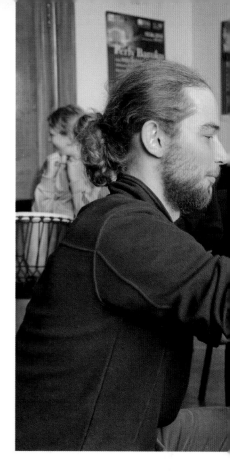

Music therapy relies on the emotive qualities of music, together with the components of rhythm, melody, and tonality, to create a therapeutic relationship. You can choose from a wide range of musical instruments, and you can even use your own voice to express your emotional and physical condition; this enables you to build a connection with your inner self, and with others around you.

Therapists combine a formal musical education and training with specific qualifications as music therapists.

Who can benefit?

Music therapy is often used when illness, injury, or disability

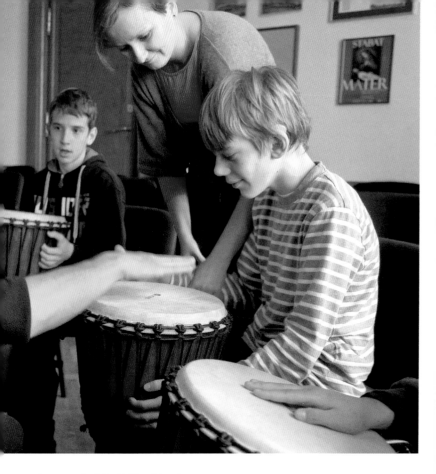

has resulted in difficulties in communication. Music therapists can work with the young and the old alike, and with a wide variety of conditions. They can evaluate and treat those who have sensory,

Music therapy is highly beneficial for children and young people who have intellectual and developmental disabilities.

physical, and learning disabilities, mental-health issues, emotional and/or behavioural problems, and neurological difficulties.

Fortunately, you don't have to have any previous musical experience or be able to play an instrument in order for music therapy to be effective.

Music therapy is most often used with:

- Children and young people, especially those with intellectual and developmental disability

- Adults with learning disabilities
- Autistic spectrum conditions
- Those living with HIV/AIDS
- Mental-health care
- Older people
- Dementia sufferers
- Neurological disability
- Victims of abuse
- Young people with eating disorders
- People with severe emotional and behavioural problems.

RESEARCH

For more than 30 years the Music Therapy Charity (see page 389) has raised funds towards research into the therapeutic benefits of music therapy. Investigations have centred on the effectiveness of music therapy with vulnerable groups, and how best music therapists can present their work.

What to expect

Individual and group sessions are provided in many different settings, such as hospitals, schools, hospices, and care homes; or, in the case of private practice, in the practitioner's office. Each session is tailored specifically to the needs of the individual, but you might reasonably expect to use accessible percussion instruments and your own voice to explore the world of sound. The music therapist will respond to your responses with improvised music. Over time you will develop a relationship with your therapist, so that you feel safe expressing and exploring your emotions.

Although every session is unique, most music-therapy sessions consist of improvisation, musical "games", and occasional use of pre-composed song. This means that the emphasis is mainly on playing music freely – making it up as you go along.

How you use the instruments will naturally reflect your emotional state at that time. The therapist acknowledges what you are expressing, and supports it with his or her own music. By playing music freely together, you and the therapist are able to form a therapeutic relationship in which communication and trust are established.

Because this relationship is central to music therapy, it is up to you whether you verbally share your feelings, thoughts, and experiences or choose to remain in silence. Be aware that sessions occasionally bring up intense and difficult feelings, but rest assured that any form of emotional expression will be accepted, and recognized, by the music therapist.

Training

There are numerous music therapists in Europe and worldwide – in the UK alone, more than 700 registered music therapists are currently practising. To find a therapist near you, look for qualified practitioners on the website of the governing body of your own country. Music therapists frequently work as members of multidisciplinary teams in health, education, or social care, as well as in private practice.

Professional music-therapy qualifications are often acquired at postgraduate level. The entry requirements are high; normally only music graduates or those with a three-year musical training leading to a diploma are accepted. If you have a degree in a different but related subject (perhaps education or psychology), you may be considered, as long as you have achieved a high standard of musical performance. Assessment of personality and suitability for the work are also taken into account at an interview.

Magnet therapy/ electromagnetic-field therapy

Magnets were used for their healing properties by the ancient Greeks, and today this therapy is gaining in popularity again, not only with the public, but also in mainstream healthcare, due to magnetic-field diagnostic techniques (such as MRI) and treatment using electrical impulses.

Magnet therapy is believed to aid the healing process by restoring the natural balance of the body as it returns a "normal" balanced charge back to each individual cell in the body. This in turn is said to stimulate the circulation, promote increased oxygen flow, and restore a normal pH value (a measure of acidity or alkalinity).

STUDY FACT

Magnet therapy is now a highly lucrative industry, with a worldwide market that is worth more than $5 billion.

Magnetic-field therapy uses magnets and electromagnetic therapy devices to combat stress, alleviate pain, and promote healing. It is claimed that the benefits range from dissolving kidney stones to aiding depression, Alzheimer's disease, and schizophrenia, and stopping hallucinations or seizures. However, the therapy is primarily used for pain relief and a reduction in bruising and swelling, especially by those who are suffering from arthritic joints.

Who can benefit?
Good scientific evidence from controlled trials shows that magnet therapy is helpful for the relief of pain from rheumatoid arthritis, sports injuries (such as

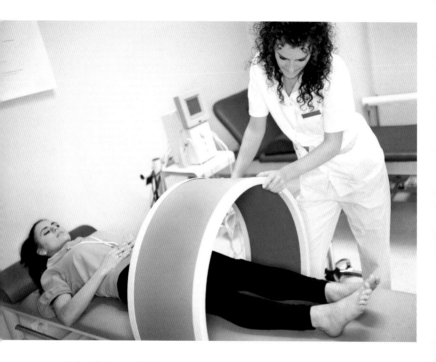

muscle bruising and joint sprains), and Post-Polio Syndrome. There is less scientific support for results for other conditions, but a great deal of anecdotal evidence exists for the following complaints:

- Fibromyalgia (a rheumatic condition)
- Peripheral neuropathy (damage to the peripheral nerves)

Electromagnetic-field therapy can relieve the pain of sports injuries, rheumatoid arthritis, and arthritic joints.

- Post-surgical support
- Lower back pain and other forms of chronic musculoskeletal pain
- Osteoarthritis
- Pelvic pain
- Menstrual pain
- Carpal tunnel syndrome

221

ELECTROMAGNETIC-FIELD THERAPY

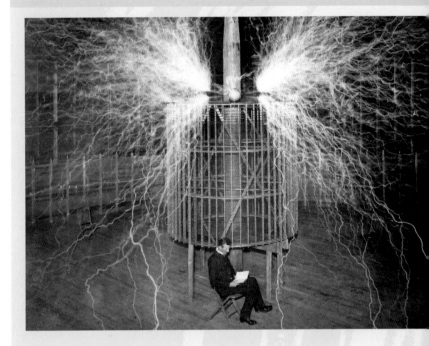

Do not confuse magnet therapy with "pulsed electromagnetic-field therapy" (PEMFT), which is used for bone-healing and, more recently, for depression.

Unlike magnet therapy, where a relatively weak static magnet is used, in PEMFT doctors apply pulses of intense electromagnetic energy to the affected area, using a special machine. In bone fractures, it is believed that the pulses bring on electrical signals at a subcellular level, which in turn encourages chemicals in the cells to repair damaged tissue.

Nikola Tesla, the pioneer of early electricity, instigated the use of electromagnetic field therapy.

Remarkably, this therapy can be traced back to the Serbian American inventor Nikola Tesla (1856–1943) – one of the pioneers of electricity use – in the early 1900s. In America the technique was initially tried out on animals, including racehorses that had broken their legs, before it was allowed to be used on humans in the 1970s.

As there is overwhelming scientific research in its favour, medics are now happy to use PEMFT for certain types of bone-fracture repair. And PEMFT for pain management, wound-healing, and depression is becoming more widely accepted.

- Sports performance – reducing muscle soreness after intense exercise
- Stress
- Headaches and migraine
- Insomnia
- Fatigue.

What to expect

Practices vary, depending on the magnet therapist, but many practitioners now use a "magmassage" – a large magnetic wand linked to an electromagnetic field – which is placed on the area of complaint for 15 minutes. In addition, individual magnets (ranging in size from small coins to large magnetic ceramic blocks) may be placed on specific areas of the body to accelerate healing.

A magnet-therapy session usually lasts around 45 minutes. Between sessions, you will be prescribed a home programme, with magnets to suit your specific needs.

Magnet efficacy and strengths

The popularity of magnet therapy has been supported by study results from the University of Virginia, which showed that by placing magnets of 70 milliTesla (mT) field strength (about ten times the strength of the common fridge magnet) near rats' blood vessels, those that had been previously dilated then constricted, and vessels that had been constricted became dilated. This implies that the magnetic field could induce vessel relaxation in tissues with constrained blood supply, ultimately increasing blood flow.

In addition, the researchers used magnets on rats' paws that had been treated, under anaesthetic, with inflammatory agents to simulate tissue injury. The magnets significantly reduced the swelling by up to 50 per cent, when applied immediately after the injury. This means that magnets could be used in much the same way as ice packs and compresses are now – for everyday sprains, bumps, and bruises, especially in sports teams and schools – with better results.

Static magnets are sold in various strengths. The units of measurement for magnet strength are gauss and tesla. One tesla is the equivalent of 10,000 gauss. Therapeutic magnets measure anywhere from 200 and 10,000 gauss, but the magnets in most common usage are 400–800 gauss.

The biggest problem for this therapy is the wide availability of cheap magnet-therapy products that enable people to self-treat; if they see no improvement, they assume it is the fault of the therapy, rather than of the magnet. Unfortunately it requires certain strengths of magnet to promote healing. Obviously magnet therapists use professional-strength magnets, but if you are self-treating it is important that you research and find the correct strength and type of magnet for the specific condition that you are hoping to heal. The type of magnets used as a self-help tool range from straps and shoes, to car-seat covers, pillows, and even mattresses.

Auricular therapy

This therapy originated in the Far East and has been practised by the Chinese for centuries as a traditional means of diagnosis and treatment. It follows the same principles as reflexology (see page 64), in the sense that a microsystem of the body exists within the ear, and stimulation or massage of those points can treat pain in other parts of the body.

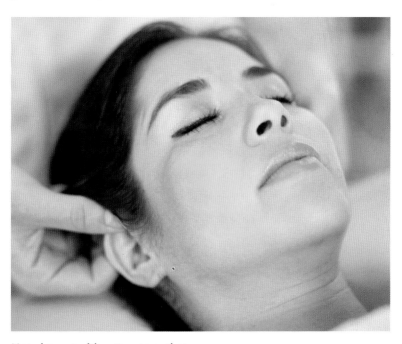

Manual massage of the outer ear can reduce pain in the corresponding parts of the body.

AURICULAR ACUPUNCTURE

The acupuncturist and physiotherapist John Tindall has pioneered the use of auricular acupuncture for detoxification and substance misuse. The therapy involves applying fine-gauge, sterilized stainless-steel acupuncture needles to five designated points on each auricle (outer ear).

Auricular acupuncture has a good track record for treating addictions and substance misuse, detoxification, insomnia, anxiety, stress management and post-traumatic stress, weight loss, emotional difficulties, and relaxation and general well-being.

Very fine needles are used for auricular acupuncture.

Who can benefit?

Anyone can benefit from auricular therapy, and it is particularly helpful if you are suffering from musculoskeletal pain, are recovering from a bone fracture, or want to lose weight without the use of medicine or invasive surgery. Auricular therapy has also shown good results among those who are attending a programme for substance or alcohol abuse, as it is helpful in improving mood levels, reducing cravings, and raising serotonin levels in the brain, resulting in a greater sense of well-being.

What to expect

Practitioners use various methods to stimulate the specific points of the ear. Some use a special probe that has a 1–2mm-long tip, to find the specific points within the ear and then to massage those points. Others rely solely on manual massage, with specific attention to the ear. Sometimes the practitioner will use acupressure pellets that are held in place in the ear by tape, to maintain continuous pressure on a reflex point; these are left attached for three to five days, to achieve effective and lasting results.

As the ear is so accessible, you do not have to disrobe during auricular therapy, which makes it quick and easy for everyone.

Training

Finding a therapist is not always easy, although auricular therapy is growing in popularity. Your best bet is to search on the Internet, but auricular therapy can also be learned readily from a basic course or reference book, and the chart and/or model is widely available.

STUDY FACT

One of the earliest uses of auricular therapy was to treat warriors and sailors in ancient China, in order to improve their vision.

THERMO-AURICULAR THERAPY

This therapy is more commonly known as "Hopi ear-candle therapy" and it is a relaxing treatment that helps those suffering from ear, nose, and throat conditions. The treatment involves placing a hollow, cone-shaped tube (candle), made of cotton that is soaked in beeswax, honey, and herbs, into the ear canal in order to stimulate points inside the ear and facilitate the removal of excess wax and impurities. The candles have a soothing effect on irritation within the ear, and can also help to ease the symptoms of sinusitis, hay fever, catarrh, excessive ear wax, tinnitus, and tension headaches. Ear-candling can also be used to instigate deep relaxation, and may be beneficial in the relief of stress and in rejuvenating the body.

Despite having been used for thousands of years all around the world, it is only recently that ear-candling has been introduced for use with conventional medical treatments, such as antibiotics and ear-syringing. However, thermo-auricular therapy is not recommended if you have grommets (a tube inserted in the eardrum to allow air to enter the middle ear), an ear infection, a perforated eardrum, or if you have had recent ear surgery.

Hopi ear-candle therapy is a soothing treatment for headaches and common ear, nose, and throat conditions.

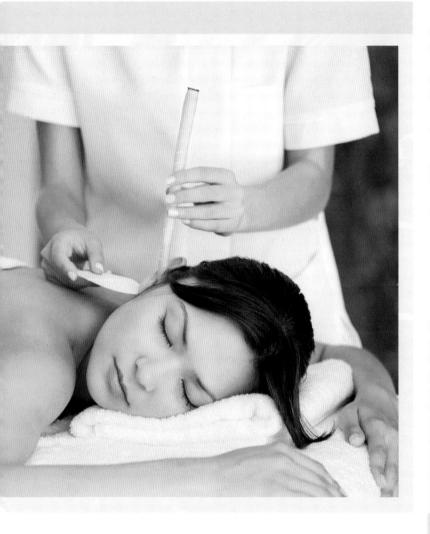

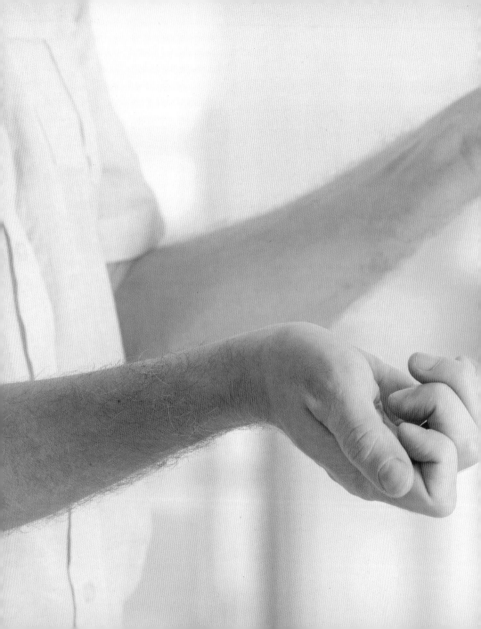

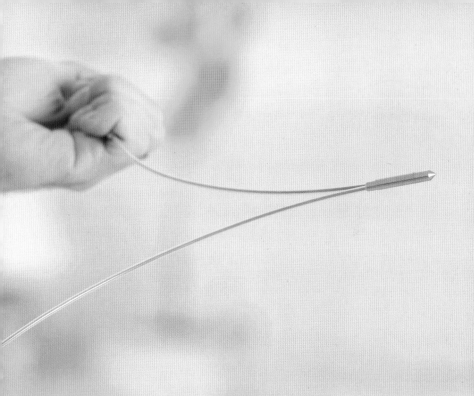

ENERGY OR VIBRATIONAL HEALING

Kinesiology

Kinesiology uses gentle muscle-testing to evaluate many functions of the body, and offers balancing techniques that can change the way you feel, effectively and quickly. Using these techniques, practitioners can get to the cause of your health problem, whether it is physical, chemical, emotional, or energetic. However, a kinesiologist does not diagnose; rather, he or she finds imbalances, and establishes what will bring the body back into balance.

Kinesiology uses specific massage points, nutrition, energy reflexes, and emotional techniques to balance you as a whole. It also enables the therapist to draw on other healing techniques and modalities and to integrate them into the session, where appropriate and as indicated by the muscle response.

History

Kinesiology was first "discovered" in 1964 by George Goodheart (see the box overleaf), an American chiropractor, who stumbled across the principle of pressure points for muscles. As time progressed, he was able to make a connection between various muscles and acupuncture meridians (see page 18). Brian Butler, who set up the first school, the Academy of Systematic Kinesiology, brought the therapy to the UK in 1975.

STUDY FACT

Applied kinesiology (known as AK for short) is a patented name in the US, while in the UK it is called systematic kinesiology (or SK), although in fact they are the same modality.

Muscle-testing against gentle pressure tells the kinesiologist about your priority stresses and how best to treat them.

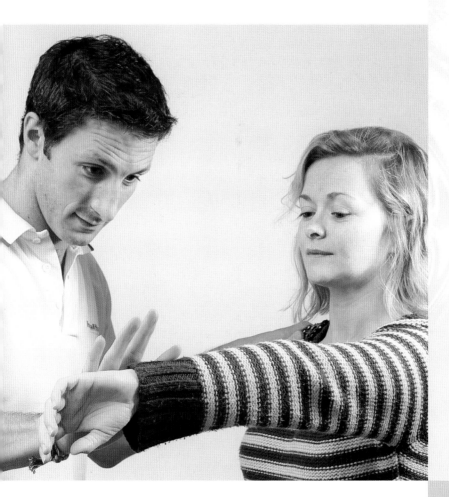

Who can benefit?

As the focus of kinesiology is on supporting the body energetically, there are many areas of your health and life that could benefit from this therapy. However, kinesiology has a recognized track record for:

- Overcoming past trauma
- Identifying nutritional excess or deficiency and allergies
- Eliminating emotional, physical, and mental stress
- Releasing fears and phobias
- Assisting with decision-making
- Improving sports performance

HEALER PROFILE

Kinesiology has its roots in the early 1960s with the American chiropractor **Dr George Goodheart** (1918–2008) who correlated the relationship between internal organs, acupuncture meridians, and skeletal muscle. He realized that the skeletal muscles (not unlike acupuncture meridians) were also a way to monitor internal function.

Muscle-testing was first developed by an orthopaedic surgeon called R Lovett to trace spinal nerve damage – weak muscles often having the same spinal nerve damage. Goodheart found that a muscle response might be affected by more than just neurological damage. Through his research, he found that there were distinct connections between muscles, organs, and the Chinese meridians of acupuncture. He gathered together a group of chiropractors interested in developing these ideas and they developed applied kinesiology and founded the International College of Kinesiology in 1973.

One of Dr Goodheart's first students was Dr John Thie, who developed Touch for Health (TFH) for lay people. He brought TFH to the UK and 60 other countries around the world. Most of the modern branches of kinesiology have developed from Goodheart's and Thie's work. Around the same time

- Enhancing learning abilities
- Aiding muscle-injury healing.

What to expect

At your first appointment, which generally lasts between one-and-a-half and two hours, your kinesiologist will take a medical and lifestyle history; subsequent appointments will last 30–60 minutes. You can remain fully clothed in a kinesiology session. The therapist will place your arm or leg into a specific position, so that the muscle is contracted, and then she or he applies light

other originators were developing their own "branches of kinesiology" worldwide, including Three in One Concepts (Gordon Stokes), clinical kinesiology (Alan Beardall), educational kinesiology (Dr Paul Dennison), PKP (Dr Bruce Dewe), wellness kinesiology (Dr Wayne Topping), and health kinesiology (Jimmy Scott). Alongside these internationally recognized branches of kinesiology there also developed a number of branches taught only in the UK, such as systematic, creative, optimum health balance, holistic, and progressive kinesiology.

Most of the established kinesiology training organizations and schools have a model of continuing professional development for instructors, and procedures for the development and inclusion of new techniques – and, with this in mind, they joined together and formed the Kinesiology Federation, which holds the recognition guidelines for upholding the highest standards for kinesiologists.

pressure against the muscle that is being tested, and you will be asked to match the pressure. This is not done to test the strength of the muscle; rather, it shows how the muscle reacts to the stimulus of added pressure: either the muscle remains in contraction or it unlocks. You should not feel any pain or discomfort during testing. Depending on how the muscle responds, the kinesiologist will then determine what the priority stresses are and the best way to address them.

The imbalances in your body are acquired in a certain order, and kinesiologists believe that you will recover more quickly if those imbalances are tackled in that order. Muscle-testing tells the kinesiologist in which order to restore the imbalances. Often, as the priority imbalance is restored, so other related imbalances vanish, too.

Using the biofeedback (the biological signals that are fed back) from the muscle test, your kinesiologist will come up with a plan of action that may include nutritional supplements,

relaxation techniques, lifestyle changes, and more. Common balancing methods may include:

- Tracing or massaging the meridians (energy channels)
- Gently rubbing, holding, or tapping acupressure points
- Gem and flower essences
- Strengthening systems with wholefood nutrition
- Sound and tuning forks
- Treatments using light and colour frequencies
- Movement, breathwork, and physical releases
- Belief-system reframing
- Clearing sabotage patterns
- Relaxation and visualization work.

Training

For membership of one of the governing bodies of kinesiology you must undergo a foundation course, followed by an advanced training course. And, once qualified, you must offer evidence of a certain number of clinical hours of practice.

CLASSICAL KINESIOLOGY AND DIVERSIFICATION

Kinesiology serves as an umbrella term for a rapidly expanding group of specialized healing modalities practised in more than 50 countries worldwide. What these different branches of kinesiology have in common is muscle-monitoring and a holistic viewpoint that honours the client's own healing process.

Classical kinesiology is based on Goodheart's original concepts, and appeals to those who prefer an orthodox approach to therapy. This system includes extensive training in anatomy and physiology, and clinical medicine, and uses a nutritional approach as well as vibrational medicine. Its therapists identify imbalances within the energy system with the aid of finger modes and biomarkers in the form of test vials. Techniques may consist of acupuncture meridian-work, gentle bone-structure and muscle corrections, emotional stress-defusion techniques, nutrition, herbs, and flower essences.

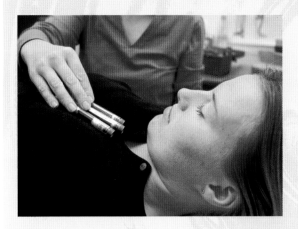

Classical kinesiologists identify energy imbalances using finger modes and biomarkers.

Angelic reiki

Angelic reiki is based on the ancient concept of angels, which is quite contrary to the popular one of today. The depiction of angels in human form with wings was popularized during the Renaissance of the 14th to 17th centuries, by artists such as Michelangelo, Raphael, Bellini, Botticelli, and Fra Angelico. Christine Core, the co-founder of angelic reiki, believes that we need to let go of the notion that angels are needed to mediate between humans and the Divine, and believes that the Divine already resides in us all.

She says, "It is only when we can let go of a paradigm which infers that human beings need something more spiritual than they are as the go-between between them and the Divine that we can truly start to embrace the concept of oneness. There really is no hierarchy in spirit.

"Angels are the messengers of God as perfect divine archetypes, based on love. Their names are a description of their particular message of truth, and their shape is the divine geometry of form. It is the study of sacred geometry which gives an understanding of the process of creation that leads to such patterns as Metatron's cube [the name given to a 3D

geometric figure composed of 13 equal circles, with lines from the centre of each circle extending to the centres of the 12 other circles].

"Creation is created according to Divine Law. The keepers and perpetrator of that law is the Angelic Kingdom of Light. Angelic reiki is the pure joy of working hand-in-hand with the Angelic Kingdom of Light."

History
Angelic reiki is the spiritual progeny of Kevin and Christine Core and, as such, holds a

In Angelic reiki, you experience how it feels to work hand-in-hand with the Angelic Kingdom of Light.

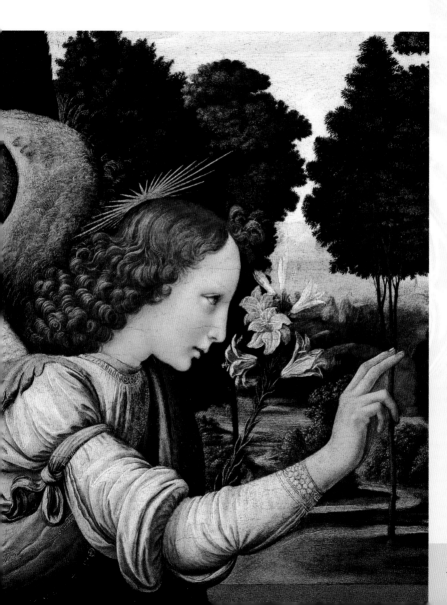

beautiful balance of male and female energy. Kevin Core channelled from Archangel Metatron the format of the healings, cleanses, and attunements; and Christine nurtured its growth, preparation for the future, and grounded it in a practical and professional way. There are now angelic-reiki practitioners in more than 23 countries around the world.

Angelic reiki is a living experience of the principle "Let go and let God", and so the master teacher does not "do" the attunements, which come directly from the angelic kingdom; he or she simply holds the space. In this sacred space

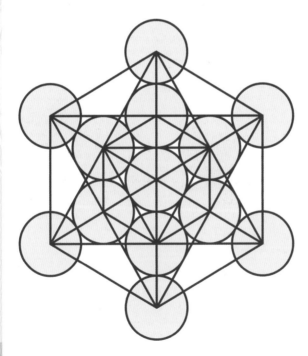

Metatron's cube is a 3-D geometric figure that is an example of sacred geometry.

each individual's healing angel presents itself energetically (you don't actually see it) and facilitates all the attunements. The angels are the only "doers" in their role as emissaries of the Divine.

Guided by angels

In angelic reiki, the whole process of healing is given over to the Angelic Kingdom of Light, where the angels reside. Christine says, "During an angelic reiki 'healing', the angels do not come to heal, improve, fix, or help; they come to remind us of the perfection that they can see and that we truly are. They fill the space that the 'healer' is holding, bringing an infusion of divine unconditional love: to hold that space is the 'healers' only purpose. They do not 'do' anything, just 'be'. No symbols to chant, visualize, or draw, and no changing of hand positions."

What to expect

"The premise of angelic reiki is that we are all perfect and loved – the practice does not look to diagnose problems, but to allow healing angelic energy to go wherever it is needed, in the belief that the healing too will be perfect for the person receiving it," explains angelic-reiki healer, Liz Dean. "Receiving angelic reiki is, of course, very personal to the recipient. Most say that they feel deeply relaxed and safe during the session; some may see colours, sense their angels' presence, or simply sleep. The recipient has no responsibility to see or do anything during the healing, other than be open to the healing possibilities that occur. The 'healer' may also see nothing, or see colours, lights, angels, sense guides/Ascended Masters, hear a message; they may see past lives of the recipient."

The session begins with a conversation with the recipient about their well-being and anything they would specifically like to address. The healing session, though, actually begins before the recipient arrives, when the "healer" does a purification visualization to prepare the space for healing, and plays music by Michael Hammer, who is a channel for the Archangel Jophiel.

The recipient lies down on a massage couch or sits in a chair. The "healer" connects with their angels and other guides, such as Ascended Masters, and asks the Archangel Michael (the most senior archangel) to preside over the healing (and to correct any mistakes, should they occur!). The "healer" makes a conscious connection with the recipient, and then begins to channel angelic energy through their hands, either touching the body on the higher heart and solar-plexus chakras (see page 176) or working in the recipient's energy field.

The angelic-reiki healer is not doing the healing, merely acting as a channel for the angelic healing energy. The "healer" is guided by their angels as to when to step back from the recipient and end the session (having set the intention to consciously disconnect); the "healer" then thanks their angels and the Archangel Michael. The healer asks Archangel Michael to ground the healing in the recipient's physical body, then shakes their hands and/or touches the Earth to send back any residual energy and to reground themselves.

Liz Dean says, "The 'healer' touches the recipient on the shoulder to tell them when the session is over, and afterwards they talk. The 'healer' is guided by their angels regarding what parts of the experience they communicate. So the 'healer' may see lots during the healing, but be guided only to discuss parts that the angels want the recipient to know."

Training

Angelic reiki is taught (by the Angelic Reiki Association, as well as by accredited practitioners) over four weekend workshops, or it can be experienced as a nine-day intensive course. The four workshops are: first and second degree; third and fourth degree; professional practitioner and service; and angelic-reiki master teacher.

Angelic reiki is not just a healing system; it offers deep

The therapist is merely a channel for the angelic healing energy.

spiritual philosophy for those who train in it, based on "The Ancient Wisdom". It also includes a broad base of information on a wide range of subjects. In the professional practitioners' workshop, valuable information is given that enables the practitioner to understand the process and purpose of the human experience of disease and healing.

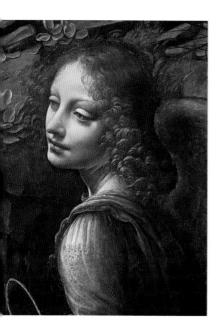

SELF-HELP

One of the chief purposes of angelic reiki is self-healing, supporting us physically and emotionally through the great changes that are being experienced at the moment. The health of the subtle body (the lowest layer of the aura, closest to the physical body) is a vital component in this process of change. Information on how this process works, and a specific healing, is given. We are experiencing many physical symptoms that are being caused by our change in consciousness. It is important for a healer to understand when physical symptoms are due to these changes and when they are caused by pathology. This information is available in the book by Christine Core entitled *Angelic Reiki: 'The Healing for Our Time'*, Archangel Metatron.

Energy medicine

"Energy medicine" is an umbrella term for most of the modalities covered in this chapter. Any healing system that works with the body's electromagnetic and subtle energies is a form of energy medicine. However, the term is also used to refer to the popular system of energy medicine that was devised, practised, and taught by Donna Eden (see the box opposite), and that is the approach described in this entry.

Energy medicine recognizes energy as a vital, living, moving force that determines much about your health and happiness. In energy medicine you heal the body by triggering its natural healing abilities, and by boosting energies that have become weak, disturbed, or out of balance. You can use energy medicine as an independent approach to self-care; as a stand-alone treatment if you visit a practitioner; or as a complement to conventional medical care. You can use it to treat physical, emotional, or mental difficulties and to promote high-level wellness and peak performance.

It is important to understand that the words "diagnosis" and "treatment" have a different meaning in energy medicine than they do in conventional medicine. In conventional medicine, you *diagnose* and *treat* an illness; in energy medicine, you *assess* where the energy system needs attention and then *correct the energy imbalances*. Physical symptoms may be a clue, but they are not the focus. For instance, the same stomach ache might trace to an imbalance in the heart meridian for one person, in the liver meridian for another person, and in the stomach meridian for a third person. The same physical symptoms can reflect different kinds of problems in your energy system, and call for different energy interventions.

HEALER PROFILE

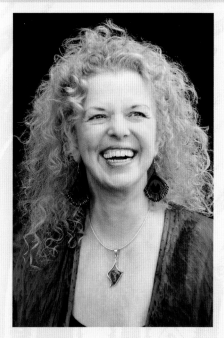

Donna Eden has perfected her own powerful form of energy medicine which she teaches in seminars all over the world.

Donna Eden has introduced her system of energy medicine to more than 80,000 people worldwide – both lay people and professionals – helping them to understand the body as an energy system. Since childhood, she has been able to see the flow of the body's energies, and from this clairvoyant ability she developed her system of energy medicine, to teach others (who do not have this gift) to work productively with the energies of their own bodies and those of other people.

Having experienced her energy medicine, I can safely say that Donna Eden is an amazing healer, and one of the most authoritative spokespersons generally for energy healing.

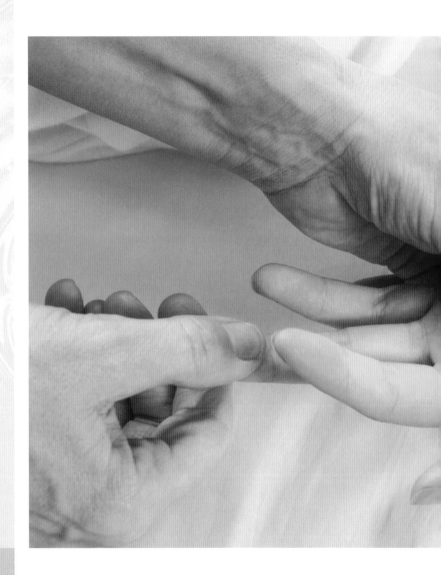

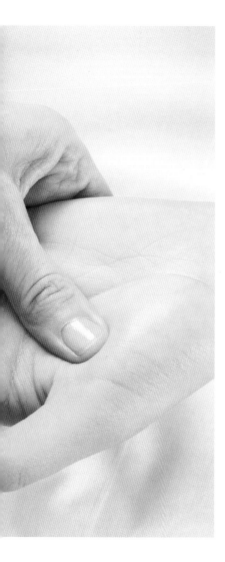

Two levels of help

Energy medicine can help on two specific levels. First, it can get the body's energies into a good flow, harmony, and balance. While not focusing on health issues directly, this can create within the body an energetic environment that supports overall health, vitality, and healing. Unlike treatments that offer pills or surgery, energy medicine focuses on the entire body as a system. Before doing more specific treatments, practitioners routinely help people get their body's overall energies into a strong and healthy flow.

Second, energy medicine involves an assessment of your body's energies and the ways in which they are related to the condition. Based on the assessment, individualized energy routines can be designed to make your energy system more robust – specifically in the ways that will help with the health condition in question.

Individual energy routines involving tapping or stimulating certain points on the body are designed to bolster the energy system.

What to expect

At your first session you will typically receive a 90-minute tracking, which determines what energy systems are out of balance and helps the practitioner to understand your unique energy system. Using techniques tailored to the contour of your energy system, you and the practitioner will begin by correcting imbalances that are in flow during the session. In subsequent sessions the systems that continue to show chronic imbalance (after correction and supporting homework from you) will become the primary focus of the energy work.

Methods used include muscle-testing to check the spin of the chakras (see page 176), the flow of energy through the 14 meridians (see page 18), the strength of the radian circuits (subtle-energy flows that support the meridians), the balance in the five-element system, the strength and function of the adrenal glands, thyroid, and reproductive systems. Wherever there is disharmony, lack of flow or strength in the system, techniques will be recommended, such as working on acupressure points; or tracing or flushing alarm points on the meridians (sometimes a blockage is found "upstream" in another meridian than the one in which the alarm point manifests), the neurolymphatics, and the neurovasculars (reflex points between the meridian and the lymphatic system and nervous

SELF-HELP

Donna Eden has devised a Daily Energy Routine (see the Innersource website on page 389) that combines the most potent techniques to help you to stimulate each of your vital energy systems and bring them into harmony and balance. It only takes ten minutes every day, but the routine can make a real difference.

system respectively), in order to restore balance.

Training

Donna Eden and her faculty, Innersource (see page 389), are committed to bringing as many people as possible to a high standard of excellence in the personal and professional practice of energy medicine. You can either follow a formal way or a less-formal, self-paced way of developing proficiency in the principles and practices of energy medicine.

The most systematic way to learn energy medicine, from the most basic principles to highly advanced methods designed for the professional practitioner, is to go through the Eden Energy Medicine Certification Program. This provides four years of training to become an energy-medicine practitioner, either with the aim of incorporating energy medicine into an existing healthcare practice, or of becoming extremely well versed in the methods for personal use. The programme is designed so that you can stop at the end of any year and still have a complete course of study. The Certification Program can be done largely at home, with four intensive four-day classes each year. The first year (the foundation programme) prepares physicians, nurses, and other healthcare practitioners and therapists to begin to incorporate energy medicine into their work.

There are other routes that do not require the level of commitment of the Certification Program, if you simply want to use energy medicine for personal use. Check out the Innersource website for instructional books and DVDs, and to find a qualified practitioner in your area.

The BodyTalk System™

Developed by Dr John Veltheim in the mid-1990s, the BodyTalk System™ presently has more than 2,000 active certified BodyTalk™ practitioners, with an estimated 100,000 clients across 40 countries, and courses in 47 countries, making it one of the larger mind–body medicine systems.

The BodyTalk System™ seeks to address the "whole person", which means that no aspect can be overlooked – be it emotional, physical, or environmental. In BodyTalk™ a whole-healthcare system has been developed that supports and promotes the well-being of any person, animal, or plant.

BodyTalk™ understands the profound influence that the psychology of the body has on our health. Instead of focusing on the symptoms, it finds the underlying causes of illness by addressing the whole person and their whole story. Its techniques provide insights to the areas of the body that require attention – what might seem like an obvious problem to you is not necessarily the one that your body wants to address first.

BodyTalk™ draws on Western medical experiences, acupuncture, osteopathic and chiropractic theory, applied kinesiology, and the insights of modern physics and mathematics.

Who can benefit?

Everyone can benefit from improving the communication within their body through a BodyTalk™ session, and it can be used as general health maintenance or to improve specific conditions, either alongside other treatments or as a stand-alone therapy.

Regardless of the diagnosis, a BodyTalk™ practitioner always focuses on the underlying causative factors. Because of this, the therapy is able to address a multitude of problems and diseases, including:

- Arthritis
- Fibromyalgia
- Hormonal issues
- Chronic fatigue
- Allergies and intolerances
- Headaches and migraines
- Digestive disorders
- Anxiety and depression
- Infertility
- Back pain
- Sleep disorders
- Asthma.

What to expect

A BodyTalk™ session takes place fully clothed and is very relaxing. After a discussion about the client's health, well-being, stresses, and concerns, the practitioner will tune into the client's body and, by using biomuscular feedback and trained intuition, builds up a picture of what the client's body would like assistance with. For example, the pituitary gland might not be communicating and synchronizing correctly with the ovaries, and this could be causing reproductive problems. In order to bring about changes, light touch and tapping over the head and sternum are used, with the appropriate focus and attention.

In terms of physics, the tapping creates a standing wave (a vibrational pattern) that creates the changes in the consciousness of the body, and this then translates into correction at all levels – physical, mental, emotional, and spiritual.

SELF-HELP

BodyTalk™ Access is a sub-system of the BodyTalk System™. In a one-day course anyone can learn a very simple and effective set of techniques to reduce stress, improve the immune system, and generally help with day-to-day health challenges. More than 26,000 people worldwide have been trained to use these techniques on themselves, their families, and their communities. There are also several outreach programmes that use BodyTalk™ Access in communities in Africa, Asia, and the Americas.

HEALER PROFILE

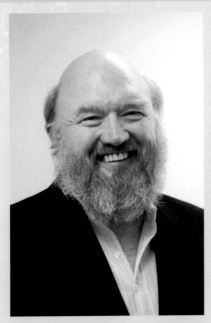

John Veltheim developed the BodyTalk System™, making sure that the practitioner's "intentions", namely their beliefs and expectations, do not inhibit the effectiveness of a session.

Dr John Veltheim's experiences as a chiropractor and acupuncturist clearly demonstrated to him that the state and quality of training of a practitioner – their focus and attention, their clarity of thought, and the rapport they have with their patients – are important factors determining the outcome of any therapeutic situation. For instance, a skilled traditional acupuncturist can effectively cause many different changes in the energy systems of the body by use of the same acupuncture point, simply by changing the intent and focus while inserting the needle.

As he began developing the BodyTalk System™, Dr Veltheim's focus and attention on the practitioner in any therapeutic situation became pivotal to his new healthcare system. In BodyTalk™ a differentiation is made between "attention" and "intention". In many energy-based therapies one hears the phrase "It is the intention that matters". However, when treatments are given with intent, the practitioner's own agenda, beliefs, and expectations can inhibit the effectiveness of the session.

Another of Dr Veltheim's requirements for the BodyTalk System™ was that he didn't want it to rely on diagnostic systems – that is, knowledge or reasoning used to diagnose a problem; first, because diagnosing rarely respects the vast complexity behind our symptoms; and, second, because it takes many years of training to be good at this, and you will always be limited by the "database", or expertise, that you have gained to date.

He realized that the body has to be looked at as a whole, and that everything within the body (in fact every cell in the body) is seen as having its own integrated energy dynamics. On top of this, great care has to be taken to consider the environmental impact of everything that is going on around the patient, as well as the patient's detailed history.

In essence, the key to lasting results is to address all the complicit, underlying factors, including biochemical breakdowns, environmental stress (family, work, toxins, and so on), genetic factors, and emotional traumas. All the basic BodyTalk™ techniques are designed with this in mind.

It was in the late 1990s that Dr Veltheim left his successful practice in Australia to move to Sarasota, Florida, in order to further his research into BodyTalk™. It wasn't long before he started to teach advanced levels of the BodyTalk System™ to others, and soon he was training other instructors in the system so that it could be taught in countries all around the world. The system is now taught in at least 10 different languages in over 50 countries worldwide.

Most of Dr Veltheim's time now is spent travelling the world and giving talks and teaching sessions on BodyTalk™ and its related wellness programmes. He still mentors and trains new instructors so that BodyTalk™ can continue to reach a wider audience around the planet.

Dowsing therapy

Dowsing involves searching for a concealed item or for hidden knowledge using a hand-held tool. In the case of dowsing for water, geopathic stress (earth energies and their effect on human well-being; ley lines), or archaeological sites, divining rods are most commonly used today (it used to be birch twigs). However, in the area of health, most practitioners use pendulums for dowsing.

As yet, there is very little scientific evidence in favour of dowsing, but it is thought that the dowsing response is probably a reaction to changes in magnetic flux in the body or in the geographic location.

What to expect

After establishing what health problems you wish to address, the dowser will set the intention and then, using the pendulum or whatever instrument they select, will ask questions and

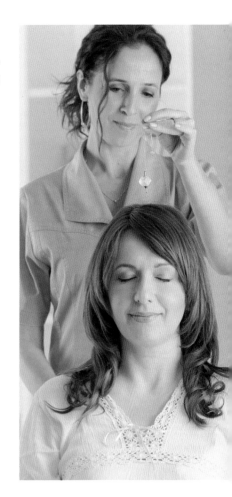

the pendulum will respond with Yes or No answers.

Many dowsers combine this skill with another modality, such as flower essences (see page 210), herbal medicine (see page 53), or nutritional therapies (see page 69). So, once the diagnosis or cause has been established, they will then dowse for the correct treatment and in what strength it should be used.

Opposite Dowsing for health-related issues usually involves the use of a pendulum or favourite crystal.

Below When divining for water, geopathic stress, ley lines, or lost items, for example, divining rods are used.

Training

There are many dowsing courses but, as with all healing therapies, it is best to go through a professional association based in your home country to find a training course that leads to a recognized qualification.

There are also countless workshops where you can learn the art of dowsing, and then you can use the pendulum or a favourite crystal or gemstone to ask about your health at any time. In this way, you can use dowsing as a self-help tool, to optimize your health, well-being, and overall quality of life.

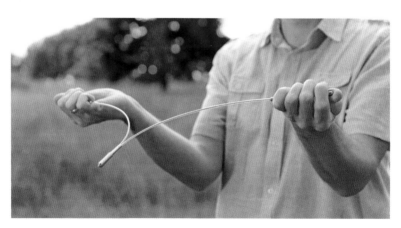

"Dowsing is the ability, latent in everyone, to discover things beyond the range of our normal five senses. Practice and use of the art in its many forms can open doorways to wider perceptions in all our experiences."

HAMISH MILLER (1927–2010), DOWSER

DISTANCE DOWSING

Dowsing can be carried out at a distance – when you are dowsing for an object, it really doesn't matter if it is in the next room or the next continent. This is extremely useful for those dowsing in the areas of earth energies, archaeology, and water services, as they can initially work from maps; but it is also effective for practitioners who dowse for health. Using a photograph, a DNA sample (such as hair), a personal item (such as a ring or an time of clothing), or a witness of the person on which to focus their attention, distance-dowsers can dowse for causative factors and suitable remedies – the latter often being found in response to a Yes or No question, or by the pendulum or the hand stopping above the relevant remedy.

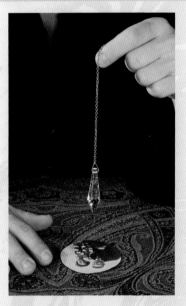

Distance divining can be achieved using a photograph or personal item, or even DNA samples, such as a lock of hair.

HEALER PROFILE

Elizabeth Brown, a dowser for more than 20 years and the author of *Dowsing: The Ultimate Guide for the 21st Century*, talks of her specialism within the field of dowser healing:

"I put forward the plea in my book for dowsing to be taken seriously in the field of health as we go down the exciting route of the amalgamation of holistic and allopathic medicine. Dowsing not only provides support for long-term health but, more importantly, it can give crucial information at the beginning when you first get a diagnosis – and this is my particular field of speciality.

"I don't diagnose the condition; you need medical qualifications to do that. As a causative diagnostician, I identify the causative, contributory, and trigger factors behind a previously diagnosed condition or a set of symptoms that has no orthodox label.

"These are all the chronic metabolic diseases. By definition, the only way to treat a chronic metabolic disease is to identify and address the underlying metabolic imbalance. And this is where dowsing absolutely excels. For someone with cancer, irritable bowel syndrome, rheumatoid arthritis, or chronic fatigue syndrome, for example, dowsing can identify the causative factors. This makes it possible to address the root causes, rather than merely treating symptoms, thereby leading to a profound change in health and preventing the likelihood of the condition returning. Treatment ceases to be a lottery and becomes a carefully tailored plan that's in the patient's best interests: one which enables them to become an active participant in their healing, and take long-term responsibility for their health. It is hugely empowering."

Zimbaté

Carolyn Snyder is a softly spoken American from Seattle who has practised reiki and other modalities for the past 25 years. However, since 2003 her priority has been spreading the word, practising, and teaching the ancient and long-forgotten healing art of Zimbaté (pronounced "Zim-bah-tay"), which translates as "A Path towards a Truth" (see the box below).

Carolyn says, "Zimbaté has been given to us by Enoch, the Patriarch of the Earth, and this is the third time. On previous occasions, the gift was abused and the energy was removed. Now, Enoch has said that mankind is ready for this gift and its responsibility. Many people, countries, and our Earth are in need of its healing rays."

STUDY FACT

As we have seen, the word "Zimbaté" can be translated as "A Path towards a Truth": note that this is *A* Path, not *The* Path. Zimbaté is an energy that is attuned to each and everyone's individuality. It is a catalyst that helps propel each of us towards our own Truth. Zimbaté recognizes that all of our paths are different, and therefore our Truths are unique.

Two main energy streams

There are two main energy streams and one is called Metatron, meaning "many diffused energies". This is the stream that reiki and similar modalities use. The Metatron vibration has been diffused so that it can be used with ease by the human body. Reiki has been the forerunner of this energy stream, and continues to provide a significant contribution to human energetic evolution.

Zimbaté comes to us from Mahatrone energy. Mahatrone can be defined as "great or celestial energy" and is a direct, unfiltered energy from the Source. With its higher vibration, Mahatrone energy is significantly more effective in vibrational tone than reiki is. And Zimbaté adds a new quality to the vibration that humans are ready to embrace and use. This means that we have a more advanced and effective tool in our spiritual toolbox.

"As I look back over 27 years of practising reiki and other energy healing modalities, it seems as if it has been leading up

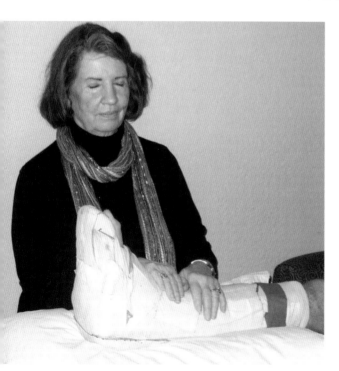

The ancient and long-forgotten healing art of Zimbaté has been rediscovered and shared by Carolyn Snyder.

to Zimbaté." explains Carolyn. "Reiki has been a great leader in the acceptance of energy work. Now the time is right to add to the foundation of reiki. Zimbaté is the most powerful energy accessible on the planet at this time. I am aware of remarkable healers who seem to defy all known healing modalities and show astonishing results, but I am referring to techniques that are teachable and are able to be passed on to others.

"Zimbaté offers another most unique gift and a source of great joy, which is the guide you will receive in your first class. Your guide will work with you any time you request their presence. You could invite your guide to help you with a client, for personal growth and understanding, or for a larger concern that encompasses a world view. The relationship is a wonderful bridge between the seen and the unseen worlds. Your guide can become an important part of your everyday life."

THE ZIMBATÉ CREED

*"I hold Zimbaté wisdom
with integrity.*

*I use Zimbaté energy
with clear intent.*

*I am mindful of
the responsibility
entrusted in me.*

*I use Zimbaté with joy
and generosity."*

Who can benefit?

Zimbaté has a broad reach and one very important distinction: it does not have any limitations. *No limitations.* Zimbaté is not limited to healing. It can be an effective tool for personal growth and spiritual evolvement. It works in – and on – the physical, mental, emotional, and spiritual realms. It is active in other modalities. Zimbaté is not limited in relation to time, space, or place. And it can be a catalyst for change. Humans are only confined by our own thinking, and how we discuss and practise Zimbaté in ten years' time could be evolved and enlightened compared to today.

"Like any practice, the more I enhance my ability to transmit, so the power of Mahatrone energy grows through me. Zimbaté is fast, clear, deep, and laser-like in its focus. It deals with the source of the issue or problem, not the symptoms. For all the power behind Zimbaté, the Mahatrone energy is gentle and soft in application," continues Carolyn.

What to expect

Your Zimbaté practitioner will be working with your own personal guide, and also with their guides. Then there is *you*: a session is all about you and your needs. You are totally in charge and will direct the energy to where it is most needed. Your human self may not necessarily be in control, but your higher self will know what is to be done. You may not always have a conscious awareness of the results, but results will occur; they may be on multiple levels (spiritual, physical, mental, or emotional) or just one level. The energy will address the predominant issue at that moment and, as we know, life is in constant flux.

A session is generally quite short, for Zimbaté is fast. Again, the circumstances can vary widely, but some clients only require sessions of 5–10 minutes to achieve the desired outcome. Many clients report experiencing positive changes and results after a session. Having experienced a Zimbaté healing from Carolyn myself, I can vouch for the power of this modality.

Zimbaté is not just for the big stuff in your life. It is for *all* parts of your life. My own experiences have shown me that there is a consistent elevation in vibration and results in my life since experiencing Zimbaté.

Training

Carolyn Snyder is a teacher and practitioner of Zimbaté in both the United States and the UK and runs regular courses (see page 389 for her website).

Divine empowerment

Divine empowerment is a new way of self-healing for modern times, which is fast, effective, and powerful enough to fit in with our permanently busy lifestyles. It was devised by Antonia Harman, and what would usually take weeks or years to learn can now be learned in a workshop in just a few minutes.

"Energy systems are a bit like iPads," says Antonia, and we can upload various "deeply nurturing energy frequencies" into our human software, just as we install apps. "Most of us are perfectly happy installing apps, and we often get excited like kids, clicking on them when the mood takes us," she explains. "Divine empowerment can do the same. In two minutes an energy app can be installed into any human system – to benefit, all we need do is click. Clicking is dead simple – say the name of the energy and then go."

In our technological age, everything is easily accessible and quick, and such rapid change makes many people feel overwhelmed. We carry a lot of stress, which not only causes misery, but can also heighten latent illness. The energies used in divine empowerment offer us the chance to experience the blessings of meditation and profound inner healing – such as "grounding" and "centring" – in just a few minutes.

Antonia Harman is the founder of divine empowerment.

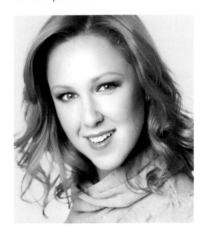

Energetic "apps"

Once you have received the energy at a workshop (just like installing an app), all you need to do is consciously call upon the energy and you will then drop into a peaceful, meditative state. It sounds too easy – too good to be true; however, according to Harman, the world has moved forward. She says, "In this crazy place, in which so many people are desperately in need of inner peace, compassion, and healing, this new programme offers a really simple and effective solution. Five minutes of passive channelling while pottering around has the effect of 20 minutes of dedicated meditation."

Harman's clients are also very happy to use "Energetic Aspirin", a natural painkiller that works within seconds: simply the intention of calling upon the energy will help you to switch out of severe pain. This "app" is also fantastic for headaches, toothaches, back pain, or menstrual cramps. During the workshop 40 or so energetic "apps" may be installed and, whether you are a veteran healer or a novice, this energy is accessible to all – to be used on yourself, your friends, and your clients.

Harman continues, "Possibly the most amazing part of divine empowerment is that the energy wants to spread, to bring light and oneness. This means that no less than 50 per cent of the energies installed at the workshop can then be taught by the students who attend." There are many other energies that can be installed at the workshop: for example, "Ying–Yang" and "Compassion", which help to clear emotional issues; "Chakra Blaster", which starts to bring the chakras (energy centres) into their true nature; and a "Tantric Meditation", which allows us to merge energetically with a partner.

What to expect

You can use the energy in three different ways:

- The first way is the traditional or "active" method, which is used while performing a healing or during meditation.

- The second way is "semi-passively": you can run energy during simple tasks such as cleaning the house, cooking dinner, or watching TV; by intention it works in the background to fit in with our busy lives.
- The third way is "passively": the energies from this system plant seeds. These seeds happily "grow on the windowsill" – which means, basically, that even if we are not actively using the energies, we are still getting the benefits from them.

After the "Introductory level", where you learn how to use energy "apps" for things such as temporary relief from pain, grounding, energizing, and emotional release, there are four more levels. These explore the Flower Of Life technology (ancient light energy), upgrading your energy body, Kundalini awakening, switching polarity, and how to heal food intolerances and allergies.

ONLINE COMMUNITY

The latest development for Divine Empowerment is an online educational community. The new website is designed to teach healing via videos. You watch a video once and the light technology embedded within it awakens your latent abilities, so you can use energy healing for yourself and others. You can join discussion groups and pose questions to Harman or fellow students, and there is unique content from her in the Vlog. The site provides content both for introductory level students – including meditation tips, instructions on how to dowse with a pendulum, and advice for removing "energetic hooks" – and for more advanced level students – including Flower Of Life work, food allergy healing, and single intention healing of various illnesses.

www.divineempowerment.co.uk/membersarea/levels

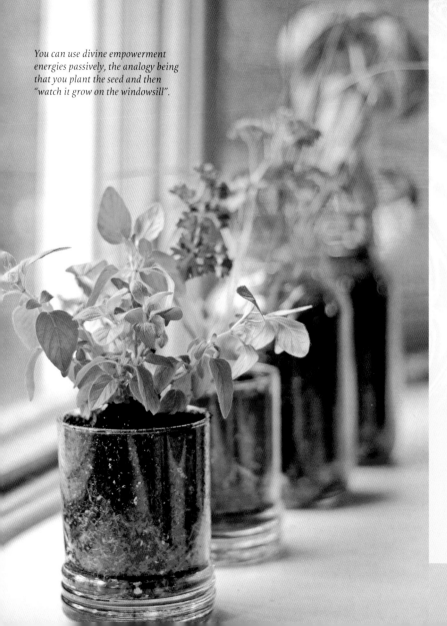

You can use divine empowerment energies passively, the analogy being that you plant the seed and then "watch it grow on the windowsill".

Metatronic Healing®

In 2007 a new energy healing system called Metatronic Healing was announced, which uses high-frequency archangelic energies to heal the heart and dissolve painful memories and outdated beliefs that might limit your life. Its founder, Philippa Merivale, has been amazed at how swiftly Metatronic Healing has taken off. She and her team run workshops and training sessions in order to train healers in this new way of working, and also give healing to those who attend.

The combination of attunements (physical touch) and transmissions (pure energy streams) works together in dynamic partnership. Each attunement is applied to an energy centre or an organ, and adjusts your energetic setting to a particular wavelength (like a radio). The attunement is followed by the transmission, which transports that wavelength into the subtle workings of your energy system, restoring the matrix of who you are as it works with you through time. A transmission connects you with the potent source of divine energy, which is the Archangel Metatron (see the box on page 268).

These shifts in your matrix are permanent: as the imprints of old wounds and destructive patterns are dissolved and removed, your original blueprint is developed, honed, and fortified. As you work through the courses (see Training, page 270), receiving deeper and deeper restoration at each stage, you also integrate more deeply than before the experiences you have gained throughout your life.

Who can benefit?

The programme of Metatronic Healing caters for a wide cross-section of needs, including those who are seeking personal healing, those who are on a path of consciousness, and those who are setting out to build a healing practice or to deepen the work they already do.

According to Merivale, "Metatron's frequencies and methods lead you towards the deep and fertile inner relationship that is vital to knowing yourself, to living in authentic power: as you let go of what doesn't work, you access more of what does. You bring more of your true, divinely-sourced Self into embodiment; you uncover your gifts and talents and purpose."

The frequencies and methods have immediate, beneficial effects, and also support you in a cumulative way through time, working with you to transform your life from the inside out.

What to expect

The core ingredients in any workshop are the attunements and the transmissions. In between those, there are group healing sessions and sharing/chat/interaction, which energetically support the process. The day often begins and/or ends with a short meditation, but each transmission tends to last 30 minutes or more (each one has its own agenda and life, and they vary according to what is happening

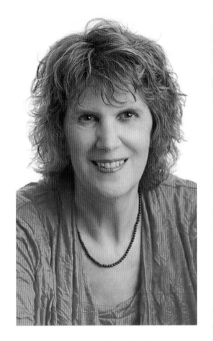

Philippa Merivale, the founder of Metatronic Healing.

in any particular group); and each transmission is preceded by a physical attunement for every attendee, so these form the main focus of the course.

On a foundation course the students are given the first "healing protocol", which means some brief practice in bringing through the

METATRON'S ROLE

In the Kabbalah – the ancient Jewish tradition of mystical interpretation of the Bible – the Archangel Metatron sits atop the Tree of Life, the ancient symbol that spans all cultures and describes the love that Divinity holds for humanity. Metatron is "charged with the sustenance of humankind", as he oversees the flow of divine energy from Kether (or the Crown) through the entire tree, or cosmos. We can interpret this to mean that Metatron plays a fundamental role in creation itself, as light steps down in frequency to become the "matter" of our material lives.

Another way of describing this role is to say that Metatron bridges heaven and earth, or the invisible and the visible. What does this mean in practice, and how does it help us as we navigate life, somewhere much closer to the bottom of that mythical Tree?

Merivale says, "Let's start from where we are: things here have grown dense, through the millennia; separation and fear have become as familiar as breathing (while paradoxically shortening the breath). The promise of Metatronic Healing is to dissolve what has kept us in fear and to awaken the intelligence of the heart, our crucial inner-guidance system. Metatron promises to reconnect us, to return us to a place where the natural energies of love, health, and joy can flow through us unimpeded. My passion and dedication are to partner with the energies of divine love, to assist in the extraordinary process of liberation and authentic, heart-based empowerment on which humanity is embarked."

The Archangel Metatron sits atop the ancient Biblical Tree of Life.

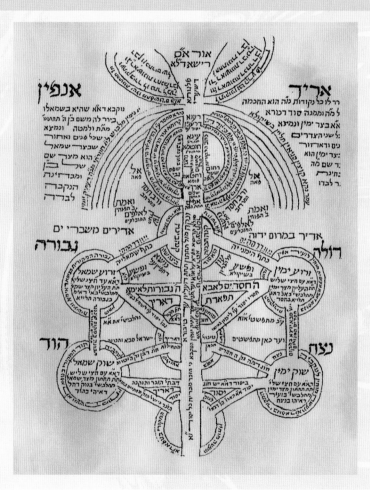

energies. Other protocols come in as students progress through the different levels of training.

A process of energetic clearance is delivered in the same manner (you are encouraged to bring a blanket and pillow, as you receive these sessions while resting in a quiet, darkened room) and dispels "the story" – or the illusions – that hold you back from real fulfilment. After a "clearance", feedback may vary, from experiencing almost a "blanking out" to vivid and powerful visions.

There are practitioner courses for those who want to practise and those who simply want personal growth.

Training

There are two practitioner courses (the foundation course and the advanced course), which run parallel to the main body of six courses for personal growth. This means that those who simply wish to take the courses for personal development can move through the six stages, from foundation ("Opening the Pathways") to "A Walk with the Masters". Those who wish to become practitioners can insert the practical courses at certain stages in that process. Full details can be found on the Metatronic Healing® website (see page 389).

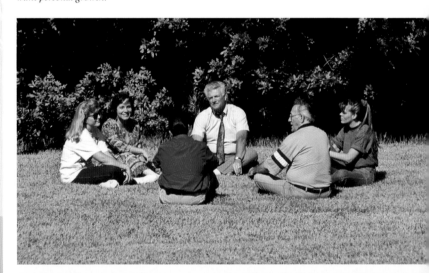

Quantum-Touch

Quantum-Touch is a simple, yet extremely effective energy-healing technique that accelerates the body's natural ability to heal itself. Widely practised in the US, Japan, and Europe, Quantum-Touch (much like reiki) uses the life-force energy inside us all – known as *qi* in Chinese or *prana* in Sanskrit – to help decrease physical or emotional pain or discomfort by means of a light laying-on of hands or by sending energy remotely. It demonstrates that consciousness affects matter and, by focusing awareness through Quantum-Touch, you can change many long-term conditions that are affecting the body and the emotions.

Breathing techniques and body-awareness exercises are used to raise the practitioner's vibration. The healer then places his or her hands on the affected area of the patient, whose body naturally raises its vibration to match the healer's, and as a result the ailment or affliction is greatly eased. This works on the same principle of resonance whereby when a tuning fork is struck, it causes another to vibrate; two people in the same energy field will naturally match their frequencies.

The founder of Quantum-Touch, Richard Gordon, says that the technique enables the

STUDY FACT

In a study that Richard Gordon conducted at the University of California, Santa Cruz, basketball players experienced an average 50 per cent reduction in their pain after the application of life-force energy, or Quantum-Touch. All 13 cases of inflammation were also significantly, and immediately, reduced.

biological intelligence of the system to do whatever healing is deemed necessary (given the right conditions), because the "spiritual intelligence", as he calls it, is smarter than we are.

Who can benefit?

As Quantum-Touch works on emotional, mental, and physical levels, it can be used to help a variety of different ailments and afflictions, to bring peace, well-being, and genuine relief from pain. It helps to release stress and emotion and accelerate healing after injury or an operation. Regular sessions of Quantum-Touch can alleviate chronic conditions such as migraine, backache, or sciatica, as well as soothe sports injuries, sprains, or aches in the body, such as frozen shoulder or pulled muscles. Devotees claim that it can also realign bones and muscle tissue that have been damaged by breaks or even by multiple sclerosis, and rebalance the emotions. Just a short session, lasting 15–30 minutes, can bring someone who is in extreme emotional distress to a place of well-being.

Everybody – from children, grandparents, and those new to (or even sceptical about) healing to doctors, chiropractors, and acupuncturists who are already treating people – can easily learn how to do this "basic human skill", as Gordon calls it, in just a couple of hours at a workshop.

What to expect

For a healing session with a Quantum-Touch practitioner you stay fully clothed and stand, sit, or lie down and relax, with your eyes closed, while the healer applies the lightest of touch to the affected area (or areas).

Every session is unique, because the areas that need work may change throughout the treatment. Many patients feel as if they are in a deep state of meditation, or as if they have suddenly fallen asleep, while the healing takes place.

Training

The quickest and cheapest way to begin learning Quantum-Touch is to do the Quantum Energy System training, an online course led by Richard Gordon, who has

HEALER PROFILE

After an atheistic upbringing, various experiences at college led **Richard Gordon** to believe in synchronicities, which pointed him towards a healer who astounded him with his abilities, and who completely changed Richard's world view. More unexplained experiences occurred and, with a desire to know what was true, Richard studied spiritual healing, therapeutic massage, and herbal medicine at the Christos School of Natural Healing in Taos, New Mexico, in the early 1970s. There he discovered the energy around his hands and began to learn how to do hands-on healing. He wrote a book on it, entitled *Your Healing Hands: The Polarity Experience*, and developed Quantum-Touch more than 30 years ago.

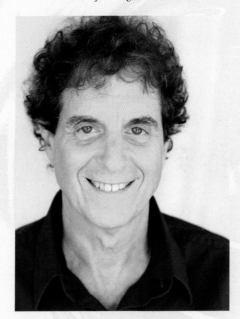

The founder of Quantum-Touch, Richard Gordon, developed the therapy more than 30 years ago.

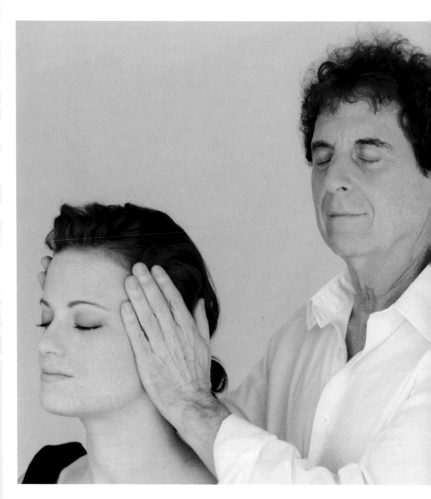

*Practising on other people is all part of a
Quantum-Touch training workshop.*

held more than 200 live Basic Quantum-Touch workshops. The course contains interactive quizzes and simple exercises to help you practise the breathing and body-awareness techniques, and various other Quantum-Touch methods. The sessions are generally 15 minutes long (sometimes longer), and show you how to heal a partner, a group, and the chakras (energy centres), among other things. These online video lessons aim to answer every question that you might ask along the way. To get the most out of them, learn faster, and receive feedback on your ability, it is worth practising with a friend, partner, family member, or even a pet.

In a training workshop to enable you to do Quantum-Touch yourself, you learn various breathing and body-awareness exercises, how to raise your energy, and you practise on the other people there. Often, even before the lunch break, attendees are raising their energy so much that they are able to reduce inflammation in others or help their bones move back into alignment, which shows how fast the results can be.

Before you can become a certified practitioner you need to complete two live Level 1 workshops, which are held in places ranging from Scotland, Holland, and France to Japan, Canada, and the US. You also need either to complete a Level 2 workshop, which takes Quantum-Touch to another level, with no limitations to your energy healing, and where you discover new and faster abilities and techniques to open to deeper intuition and heal even more (including trauma); or you must do a Self-Created Health live workshop or teleseminar, which it took Richard 29 years to develop, and which explores the emotional causation of illness and how to transform it with love. On this course people move from emotional and physical suffering to profound forgiveness and an understanding of our infinite loving nature, which can heal everything.

Chakra healing

According to many Eastern philosophies and healing practices, the chakras are spinning spheres of energy that run in a vertical line in the body, from the base of the spine up to the top of the head. These energy centres spin at different frequencies, and when they are at the correct frequencies all systems of the body work properly, so our emotions are balanced, we feel relaxed, and are in optimum health.

If any of the chakras don't spin at the correct frequency – being either too fast or too slow – we can become unwell or start to feel fatigued, depressed, or imbalanced in some way.

Healing the chakras regularly, through meditation, massage, aromatherapy, and many other daily activities (such as regular exercise and eating nutritious food), helps to keep their energy flowing well, ensuring that we stay emotionally and physically at our best.

Since the paradigm "shift" of 2012 (see page 9), some therapists now also work with higher chakras that exist in the energy field, as well as with the seven previously known chakras around the body.

History

The concept of chakras comes from Hindu culture, which dates back more than 5,000 years. Much of what we know about the chakras comes from the Upanishads, the sacred writings from the Hindu scriptures that are as known as the Vedas. The Brahma Upanishad describes four places where the soul dwells, and from where different types of consciousness arise: the naval is waking consciousness; the heart is dreamless sleep; the throat is dreaming consciousness; and the head is the transcendent state. Tibetan, Indian, and other traditions following on from this regard the chakras as centres of consciousness, which you can tune into in order to develop increased awareness.

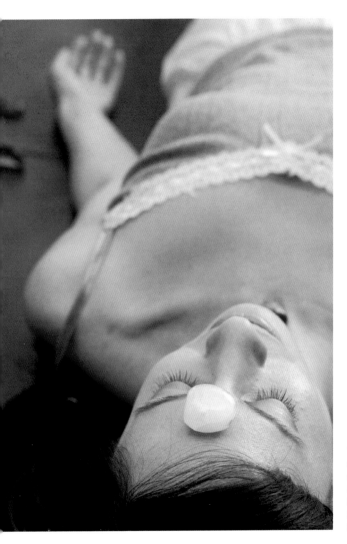

The placement of appropriate crystals on the chakras is a common tool that is used in chakra healing.

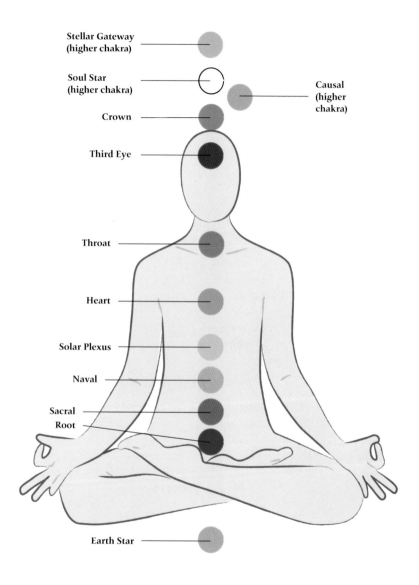

Stellar Gateway
(higher chakra)

Soul Star
(higher chakra)

Causal
(higher
chakra)

Crown

Third Eye

Throat

Heart

Solar Plexus

Naval

Sacral
Root

Earth Star

Much of the West's understanding of the chakras comes from theosophy, the school of mystical thought that was begun in 1885 by Madame Blavatsky. The theosopher Charles Webster Leadbeater travelled with Blavatsky around India in the late 1880s and wrote *The Inner Life* (1922) and *The Chakras* (1927). He believed that by tuning into your psychic intuition, you can see the chakras as rotating discs or vortices of energy. He was the first person to suggest that the chakras transform energy, and to link the various layers of the aura (the subtle-energy that surrounds the body), including the mental, etheric, and astral layers.

Writer and theosophist Alice Bailey also associated the chakras with certain endocrine glands, such as the pineal, pituitary, and thyroid glands, which are located in the same place as the chakras.

Since the paradigm shift of 2012, healers have been working with higher chakras that exist in the energy field in addition to the seven previously used body chakras.

Who can benefit?

Potentially everyone can benefit from chakra healing, but as each of the seven chakras represents different emotions and functions of the body (relating to its position), you need an understanding of the different associations to work out which chakra treatment might be of benefit in a particular case:

- **THE ROOT CHAKRA** (seen as red) sits at the base of your spine and governs your basic survival needs and physical body. When it is out of balance, you experience worries about providing for yourself or not feeling supported. Physically you may have issues with the lower half of your body, such as knee pain, arthritis, constipation, or sciatica.

- **THE SACRAL CHAKRA** (orange) is located 5cm (2in) below your navel and guides your sexuality and sensuality. When this chakra is imbalanced, you may have hip, pelvic, and lower-back pain, sexual or reproductive issues, or addictions. Emotionally you might fear commitment in your relationships, due to betrayal, past hurt, or impotence.

• **THE SOLAR-PLEXUS CHAKRA** (yellow) is located at the bottom of your ribcage. If it is blocked, you may have problems with your digestive system, liver,

or pancreas (such as diabetes), or chronic fatigue, high blood pressure, or stomach ulcers. If you have low self-esteem, energy, or confidence, then this chakra is also imbalanced.

• **THE HEART CHAKRA** (green) covers physical conditions related to the heart and upper

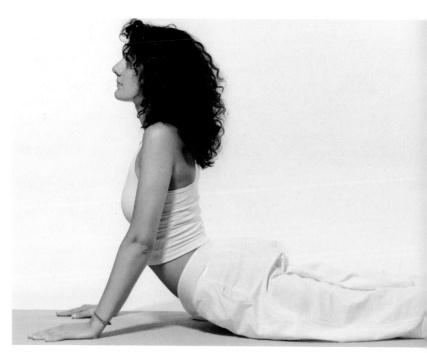

chest, such as asthma and heart and lung issues, as well as upper-back and shoulder problems. Obviously this chakra governs the emotions of the heart, so if it is not working well you may feel angry, bitter, or jealous of partners, instead of joy, compassion, and love in your relationships.

- **THE THROAT CHAKRA** (blue) needs to flow with energy or you will experience sore throats, ear infections, neck and shoulder pain, as well as issues with communication – ranging from stuttering and silence, to saying too much.

- **THE THIRD-EYE OR BROW CHAKRA** (indigo) is located between the eyebrows and will cause headaches, blocked sinuses, and eye issues if it is blocked. Imagination, intuition, and insights come from this chakra, so if any of these areas are stifled – if you're feeling moody, volatile, or unfocused – this is a good chakra to unblock.

- **THE CROWN CHAKRA** (violet), on top of the head, governs our connection with and understanding of the Divine, so if it is not functioning properly, you may experience rigid thoughts concerning religion, confusion, or depression.

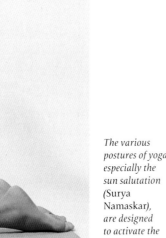

The various postures of yoga, especially the sun salutation (Surya Namaskar), are designed to activate the chakras.

What to expect

Various treatments help heal the chakras, bringing you into balance emotionally and physically – including yoga, where the different postures of the Sun Salutation pose activate each chakra; and reflexology, where areas on the feet corresponding to the chakras are massaged to get the energy moving. Crystal-healing, lying down fully clothed, with different crystals placed along the front of your body in the positions of the chakras, is another treatment that might help to heal all the chakras. Some practitioners are now using the new high-vibration crystals that have been discovered in recent years, and which are believed to help us with the "new age" of elevated awareness that we entered in 2012.

Alternatively, you can follow a guided meditation such as Doreen Virtue's *Chakra Clearing* CD (which is available from Amazon, or downloaded as an app through iTunes), which uses colour visualization to clear clogged chakras.

To heal specific chakras, try the following:

- For healing of the root chakra, connect more with your body through sports, dance, or massage; try gardening or pottery to feel more grounded.
- The sacral chakra will also benefit from dance, and from connecting with your senses through sound, music, and food.
- To help heal the solar-plexus chakra, do sit-ups to support the area, try martial arts to bring physical confidence, and undertake psychotherapy for emotional strength.
- The heart chakra can be boosted by doing breathing exercises, as well as by writing down in a journal your feelings about your relationships.
- An imbalanced throat chakra can also be helped by journaling. Use your voice more, by singing, chanting, or shouting, if you need more energy in this area; or take time to sit in silence and

Massage is another way in which to balance and heal particular chakras.

listen to others, if you have too much energy. Neck and shoulder massage, or Pilates to stretch out aches and pains in the upper back and neck, will also help.

- To unlock your third-eye or brow chakra and free up your imagination and intuition, try painting and drawing – seeing what emotions emerge afterwards, for extra insight into your situation. Studying your dreams, and meditating regularly will also connect to your deeper intuition.

- To keep the crown chakra clear, meditation is essential. If you have weak energy in this chakra, you need to open your mind to spirituality; whereas too much energy here means that you need to become more grounded in your body, by doing more physical exercise.

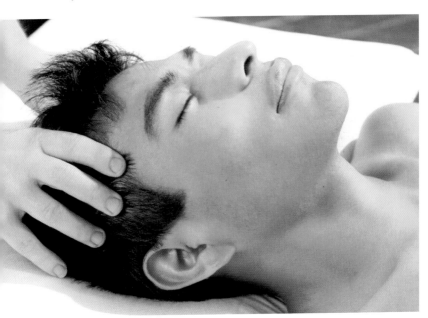

The Journey

Pioneered by international bestselling author and mind–body healing expert Brandon Bays, following her own journey of self-discovery (healing from a basketball-sized tumour in just six-and-a-half weeks), The Journey is a life-transforming therapy, which you can use in every area of your life to uncover and awaken your limitless potential.

The scientific community has proven that every emotion has a corresponding chemical that is released into the body during times of stress, trauma, or highly emotional experiences. If we suppress these emotions, then the chemicals get stored inside the body and, over time, lead to emotional and physical blocks, limitations, and even illness. The Journey is used by hundreds of thousands of people worldwide, from all backgrounds, regardless of age or culture. It enables you to get to the root cause of what is holding you back and creating disease in the body, by clearing emotional blocks and memories stored in your cells. In this way you can restore the body's natural ability to heal.

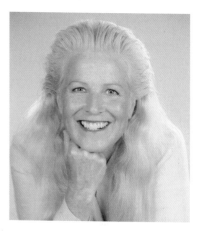

Brandon Bays, the founder of The Journey.

Who can benefit?

All over the world, hundreds of thousands of people – including children, government officials, medical professionals, and teachers – have experienced this powerful, repeatable, down-to-earth method of clearing physical ailments, emotional issues, and relationship or career problems. Whether your issue is a persistent mental or physical health one that you'd like to be free of, feelings of paralysis or depression, fatigue, anxiety, stress, or procrastination, or you long to discover and live your true purpose with passion, then The Journey could be for you.

What to expect

The first step is the three-day Journey Intensive and Advanced Skills workshop, on which you get direct experience of this liberating work. Partnering with like-minded people, using cutting-edge tools and process work, you will uncover the blocks that are holding you back in life, let go of long-standing issues, and forgive, opening the door to healing. Partnering others in their healing is powerful and creates lifelong friendships and ongoing support. With live demonstrations and teachings, you will learn step-by-step the transformational tools that can bring forgiveness, lightness, and joy into your life.

UNBLOCKING "DIS-EASE"

The Center for Disease Control and Prevention tells us that 85 per cent of all illness is due to emotional issues. The Journey works because scientists and medical doctors, such as Dr Bruce Lipton, Dr Candace B. Pert, and Deepak Chopra, MD, have proven that repressing emotions leads to individual cell-receptors becoming blocked, which leads, over time, to "dis-ease". If we address these blocks, then all healing is available: emotionally, physically, and spiritually.

Throughout the event you will be supported by a team of Brandon's staff, Journey-accredited practitioners who have undergone in-depth, year-long training with Brandon, and Journey graduates, who have vast personal experience of using Journey-work on a daily basis to clear their own issues and facilitate others on their own journey to freedom. Workshop clients constantly report amazing healing stories, experiences, and breakthroughs with issues that have been with them for a very long time, ranging from depression to anxiety, low self-esteem to feeling unloved – in fact, any and all emotional and physical issues.

Once you have completed The Journey workshop, you are eligible to attend the Manifest Abundance retreat, the first course of the life-transforming Practitioners' Programme. Here you uncover the silent saboteurs: beliefs and patterns that are keeping you from living abundantly in all areas of your life.

Next comes Brandon's favourite seminar, the eight-day No Ego retreat, for those wanting to live in complete freedom by penetrating the lies, core beliefs, and patterns that they have mistakenly believed to be who they are. This liberating retreat deconstructs the false scaffolding of the ego, uncovers what is really driving your unique patterns of behaviour, and, ultimately, leaves you soaring as your true essence, living an open, authentic life, free from self-sabotage and imposed limitations.

STUDY FACTS

Since 2008 the government of the Netherlands has sent employees to undertake The Journey to help them recover from stress and burn-out. Staff from 12 governmental departments, as well as other institutions and companies in the country, have recovered quickly, with almost no cases of relapse.

The Journey workshops and advanced retreats are now held in 44 countries worldwide, and Brandon Bays's first book, *The Journey*, has been translated into 23 languages and has sold more than one million copies.

Training

If you have a deeper thirst, you can find more information on The Journey website (see page 390), which guides you through all the seminars on offer. The Journey Accredited® Practitioner Programme is a seven-part series of courses, designed to heal your life and help you to make the same transformation possible for others.

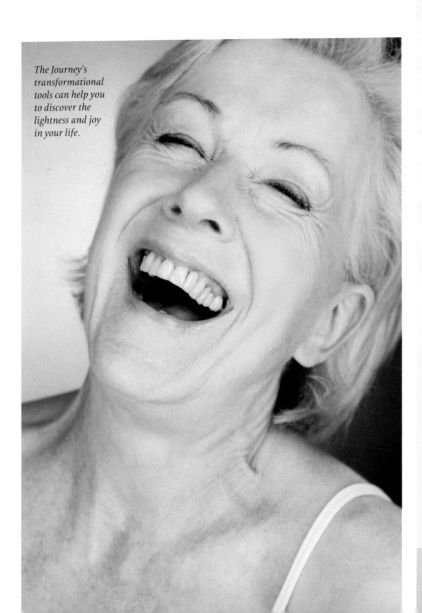

The Journey's transformational tools can help you to discover the lightness and joy in your life.

ThetaHealing®

Created by Vianna Stibal in 1995, ThetaHealing® is a spiritual philosophy technique based on focused thought, prayer, and meditation, which is practised to induce theta brain waves – the relaxed, spiritual, subconscious level of brain waves, thought to be experienced only when sleeping or in deep, yogi-level meditation. By tapping into these theta waves using Vianna's techniques, you can connect with the Creator of All That Is/the Source/God to identify issues, limiting beliefs, and illnesses, and to enable healing of the body and emotions to happen spontaneously.

ThetaHealing® works on the mental, physical, and spiritual levels of your being to teach that you are a part of God, and how to connect to this power to create change in your life. Its seven Planes of Existence concept enables you to connect to the highest level of love and energy of All That Is, for maximum clarity, wisdom, and love in your life.

This therapy is most famous for its four-level belief and feeling work, which empowers people to remove negative subconscious beliefs that are sabotaging their lives, and replace them with positive ones that can bring success and enlightenment.

By working on your core, gene, history, and soul levels of beliefs, you can change how your mind influences your body and achieve optimum health.

Who can benefit?

Although there is no need to be religious for ThetaHealing® to work, it helps to have a belief or faith in a creative spirit behind everything – the power of God, if you like. But ThetaHealing® can benefit anyone from any walk of life, whatever their age, race, or religion.

ThetaHealing® techniques can connect you to the Source/God.

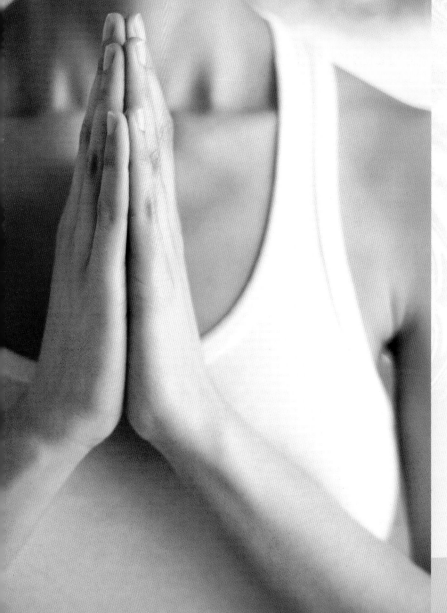

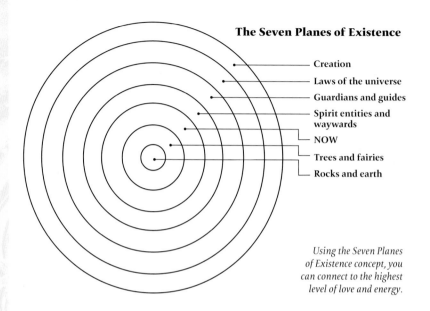

The Seven Planes of Existence

- Creation
- Laws of the universe
- Guardians and guides
- Spirit entities and waywards
- NOW
- Trees and fairies
- Rocks and earth

Using the Seven Planes of Existence concept, you can connect to the highest level of love and energy.

Whether you are sick, tired, lonely, or just feel the need to help others and improve our planet, then ThetaHealing® could be right for you to bring about the change you desire, using some simple techniques. If you feel the urge to connect to your intuition, to the Divine Spirit that connects us all, and see real improvement in your own or others' well-being, then this therapy would be a good one for you to try.

What to expect

Anyone can learn how to do ThetaHealing® for themselves from Vianna's books on the subject (see the website address on page 390), or by going to one of her many seminars that are held all around the world. If you want to become a practitioner yourself, you should do a class so that you have other people to practise on and give you feedback, and you will get to

HEALER PROFILE

Already a naturopath, massage therapist, and intuitive channel, **Vianna Stibal** discovered in 1995, during readings for other people when she tuned into her higher intuitive power, that she was also able to heal her clients. When the mother of three was told she had cancer of the femur, she tried conventional and other alternative medicine, but to no avail. Then she used this technique to heal herself and, miraculously, it worked.

Wanting to understand the background behind her method, Vianna invited a physicist to find out. Using an electroencephalograph, they discovered that her meditative healing tapped into theta brain waves, and so ThetaHealing® was born. Vianna initially started teaching it to find out if others could perform it too, which they could. She now holds teaching seminars all around the world, showing thousands of others how to do ThetaHealing®; and she has trained practitioners who are now working in 25 different countries, and even doctors in hospitals are trialling the technique.

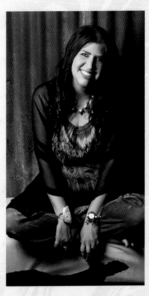

Vianna Stibal is the founder of ThetaHealing®.

learn from the originator of the technique herself.

The Basic DNA three-day event covers everything already mentioned, introduces ThetaHealing® meditation and prayer techniques, and focuses on activating the DNA that is within us all. It is believed that DNA not only carries the blueprint for our physical and psychological make-up, but also our emotional and behavioural patterns. In ThetaHealing®, DNA activation can recode any dysfunctional or harmful traits and clear any negative genetic inheritance – that is, you will find out how to identify the deep, subconscious beliefs and emotions that you have inherited from your ancestors, and how to replace them with positive ones and do the same for other people. Through this you will learn how to balance your moods, how to work with guides and angels, and the power of connecting to the Source.

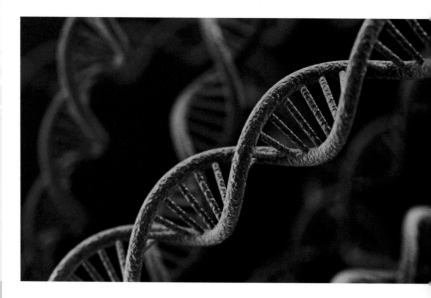

Training

Once you have participated in the Basic DNA course, you are ready to become a ThetaHealing® practitioner, if you wish. But with many more events and workshops on offer, covering more specific areas of the healing modality, you may wish to do a few more courses to become truly proficient and experienced in helping others.

The Advanced DNA sessions build on what you have learned from the Basic DNA course and add an in-depth exploration of the seven Planes of Existence that surround us, to bring you self-acceptance and appreciation of the present moment. After attending the two DNA courses, you can then move on to the Soul Mate workshops, to clear any fears and negative beliefs that you may have concerning finding your soulmate and opening to true love – whether you are in a relationship and wanting to reignite the spark, or single and trying to attract a partner.

Other courses include Intuitive Anatomy and Disease and Disorder, where you learn more about the systems and organs of the body, and how disease is created and healed; Animal seminars, for potential animal healers; and Manifesting and Abundance, where you learn to clear self-limiting beliefs about yourself, to bring about success and happiness. There is also a full range of instructor courses in all of the various seminars, so that you can teach others the ThetaHealing® technique; and higher levels of qualification include the Master Certification and the Certificate of Science. All of these are available through the ThetaHealing® website (see page 390).

Activating the DNA is part of the practice of ThetaHealing®.

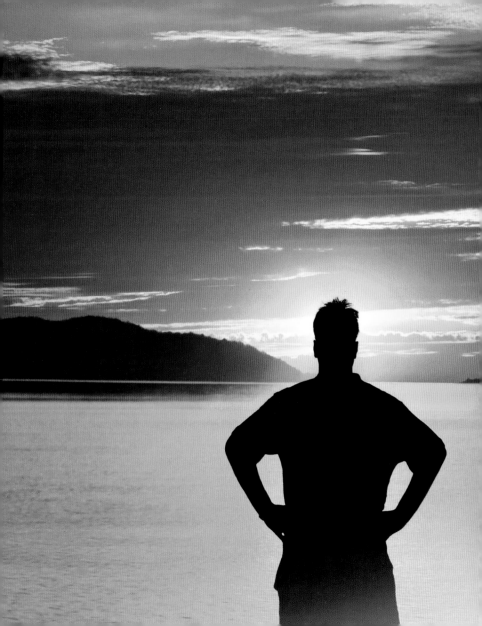

PROGRESSION AND REGRESSION THERAPIES

Past-life regression therapy

Past-life regression is a therapy that is used to help you to access hidden memories in the subconscious mind, by taking you back through previous lives. A trained therapist will lead you, using hypnosis and visualization procedures that are similar to those used in some forms of meditation.

People go for past-life regression for a variety of reasons; for some, it is merely due to curiosity about who they might have been in previous lives. But for most people it is a path for personal growth and healing. With the help of a trained guide, past-life regression can help you to:

- Understand personal relationships
- Energize talents and abilities from the past
- Release fears and anxieties linked to past-life traumas
- Release past-life traumas at the root of physical problems
- Understand and align with your life purpose – for instance, why you are drawn to certain places or have a particular interest in something.

CAUTION

Past-life regression can be a very powerful tool in accessing unconscious material. Just make sure that you consult a trained and experienced past-life regression therapist who is able to guide you through, and take some responsibility for what happens, when you start exploring the unconscious.

Your past-life experiences can be at the root of physical or emotional problems in this life.

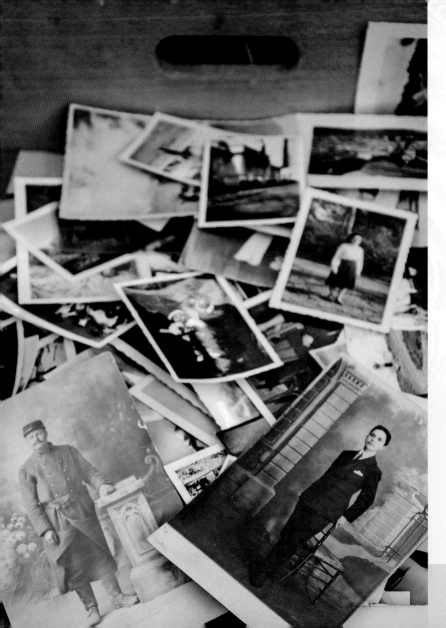

What are past-life experiences?

There is no definitive answer as to what past-life experiences may be. However, the most common theories are:

- **REINCARNATION:** The belief that we return to this world many times in order to experience and evolve.

- **GENETIC MEMORY:** Some people believe that our memories are passed on from one generation to another through the body's cell structure or DNA.

- **SOUL MEMORY:** Others believe that we can access the memory of another soul through the Akashic Records (see page 310) – the spiritual record of everything that has ever happened.

- **IMAGINATION:** It's not uncommon to find yourself wondering whether these "regressions" are in fact just figments of your imagination. Supporters of past-life regression therapy argue that countless cases can be documented through historical research, which prove the accuracy of the information, far beyond the chances of random imagination.

Who can benefit?

The person that you are today is the sum of all the experiences you have had over previous lifetimes. Past-life experiences shape certain aspects of your behaviour today and, in some cases, past emotional traumas can cause psychological problems, which cannot be resolved using normal psychotherapy. Using past-life regression, a therapist can help you to release repressed thoughts

STUDY FACT

Past-life regression therapy should not be confused with a *past-life reading*, which is a passive process and has little therapeutic effect.

and affect a valuable change. You may be surprised at what comes out of a session. Many people believe that re-experiencing and processing a past-life memory may help you to understand and resolve current relationships, begin to untangle emotional problems (including phobias and compulsions), and even heal physical complaints.

What to expect

A past-life regression therapy session typically lasts between two and three hours. After an initial interview – during which you may discuss why you want to do the regression, what you hope to achieve from being regressed, and a few details about your current life – the session starts.

While in a light trance, you experience each past life yourself. You see it, sense it, and feel it. You are the central character deeply involved in the past-life story, and the therapist may ask questions, which you answer as you progress through the session. The regression itself usually lasts 60–90 minutes, and you may

experience up to three lifetimes during that period.

After the regression, the therapist will allow you time to talk about the experience. You may feel peaceful and a little "spaced out", or even somewhat drained and disoriented. These are all common reactions to past-life regression.

RELATIONSHIPS

Quite often relations, friends, and even rivals in this lifetime are in fact groups of interacting souls who reincarnate together. Some believe this phenomenon happens to balance the laws of karma – that is, the harmony or disharmony caused by people's behaviour towards each other. Perhaps you meet someone for the first time and feel you have known them all your life; interacting soul groups could be the reason, and a past-life regression session might help you discover these individuals.

Past-life integration therapy

Past-life integration (also known as Soul Wisdom healing) is a therapy that consists of four steps through which a past-life integration (PLI) therapist will teach you how to free yourself from destructive thoughts, feelings, and behaviours, which is a valuable tool for life.

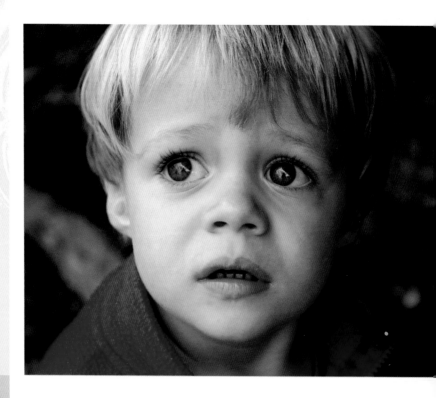

Past-life integration therapy is based on the theory that, as adults, we often perceive the world through the defence mechanisms that we developed as children. These defence mechanisms make sure that we do not have to feel the pain that was inflicted upon us as children, but they are exactly what make us suffer most as adults. They give us a distorted view of the present reality.

You may well have genuine problems today, but anxiety, depression, insecurity, stress, anger, addictions, and relationship conflicts can also be defences used as protection against pain from the past. PLI helps you to become aware of just how you became entangled in these defences and how to dismantle them. It can profoundly change your world and your relationships.

The aim of PLI therapy is not to feel the old pain, in order to do some work on it so that it goes away, but rather to live your life increasingly free of defences. It helps you to recognize when a defence is being activated, so that you can dismantle it more effectively and more quickly each time. Eventually you can eliminate the destructive effect of it in your daily life.

History

The Iranian-born Dutch psychologist Ingeborg Bosch started the work of past-life integration therapy, and it then grew into a coalition of independent, qualified

STUDY FACT

The content and application of the cognitive, behavioural, and emotional elements of past-life integration therapy is very specifically defined and is unique to PLI. It should not be confused with any combination of other cognitive, behaviour, and regression therapies.

Overcoming the defence mechanisms that we develop as children is at the core of past-life integration therapy.

professionals in increasing numbers (all of whom are driven from the heart), who practise past-life integration therapy all over the world.

Apart from giving therapy and writing books, Bosch is dedicated to the training of therapists in order to make past-life integration therapy more and more accessible to the wider public.

Who can benefit?

PLI therapy can be useful in the treatment of conditions such as:

- Depression
- Addictions
- Education issues
- Panic attacks
- Fear of failure
- Aggression
- Anxiety about public speaking
- Weight issues
- Jealousy
- Social phobias and friendship issues
- Grieving and loneliness
- Issues concerning sexuality.

What to expect

The number of sessions that is required varies from individual to individual, but past-life integration therapy is a moderately lengthy process and you should reckon on at least 20 sessions initially.

The first phase of PLI is based on Self-Observation (cognition).

SELF-HELP

In her latest book, *Past Reality Integration: 3 Steps to Mastering the Art of Conscious Living*, Ingeborg Bosch presents PLI steps that you can practise at home in order to change your life. The self-help steps are presented in three phases and take nine weeks in total to complete. Bosh has developed lots of practical self-help tools, such as the Personal Defence Profile Test, the Defence Recognition Test, and Self-Observation forms, which you can download and print out.

By observing yourself closely, you will come to recognize when you are behaving defensively. Soon you will learn to distinguish between the adult consciousness and the child consciousness – namely, whether the feelings are caused in the here and now or whether they are old.

Phase two is known as the Defence Reversal (behaviour) phase. Once you are able to recognize your defences, you can then start reversing them each time they are activated. Occasionally during this phase you might be invited to explore "exposure", when you deliberately expose yourself to the very things that you would most like to avoid, in order to gain access to the feelings that are hidden by your avoidance of them. This phase will help you to acknowledge that you do not need to defend yourself any more.

Phase three is all about Regression (emotion). The therapist will teach you to use regression yourself – however long that might take. It is important to be able to do this, so that you can connect old pain to its true cause, or the old reality. Once you are aware of what the old repressed reality looks like, and you know on an emotional level what it would have felt like, it is no longer necessary to experience the same old pain over and over again whenever a trigger is confronted.

In the final phase, known as Dual-Consciousness (cognition, behaviour, emotion), you are able to notice when you feel old pain coming up and identify it as such; know what the Symbol is, recognize the pain that the Symbol brings up, and which old reality it is connected to; allow the pain to be in your body, without suppressing or defending against it (as you would have done before PLI therapy); and stay connected to the present reality, so acting according to your adult consciousness as opposed to your defences. Once you have reached this fourth phase, the three pillars of PLI – cognition, behaviour, and emotion – integrate into one.

Future-life progression

Future-life progression (FLP) is one of the latest techniques to take the healing world by storm, and leading FLP practitioners are being consulted by everyone from governments, major corporate companies, and research units to movie stars and the military.

FLP was discovered in 1977 by the American hypnotist Bruce Goldberg. He found that by going into a hypnotic or relaxed state, you can see your future, months or years down the line. This is not clairvoyance, because the client does the work himself or herself, through a deep meditative state.

Who can benefit?

FLP practitioner Lorraine Flaherty, who is also a trained hypnotist, says, "FLP gives you choices with regards to how you live your life now, and gives you an idea of how your actions and thoughts in the now will affect your future. You are in control."

Aspects of serious illness and death are not subjects that any

Lorraine Flaherty is a leading future-life progression practitioner.

responsible practitioner will delve into. FLP is used for practical topics, such as work, relationships, home, and other things that we can improve on. A session is designed to show people what their "most probable" future will be, if they stay on the same path without making any changes.

Lorraine says, "This is really a very common-sense idea, but many people do not take the time to think about the consequences of their choices and actions. Stepping into this version in the session provides a complete reality check. People then get to explore alternative versions of their life – focusing on specific ideas that they may have in mind – and perhaps some that they hadn't even thought of.

"The best part is taking them into the highest potential version of their future, so they get to see what they are really capable of. This can really inspire people to want to do more with their lives, and gives them motivation to make the changes that are required. The outcome of this is that people leave with a greater sense of direction, they gain the ability to focus on what is important to them as they move forward in their lives, and this reduces the stress from all decision-making. Knowing where they are headed leads to peace of mind and greater inner confidence."

So what about karma – the law of cause and effect? Is it right that we can circumnavigate events from which we should perhaps be learning, in order to take us to a different place next time round?

Flaherty says, "People still have choice over whether they make the changes suggested, and clearing karma is all about making better choices; any help that can be offered with regard to helping it along can only be a good thing. I think that right now we, on the planet, are at a place where we need to clear our karma, and I think that techniques like past-life regression and the future-life work are providing opportunities for people to do just that; by clearing away the unnecessary mental clutter, and creating more balance in our lives, we can raise our vibrational energy and make way for more light and love to come in.

"You can also use FLP for looking at the state of the planet, the economy, world peace – it works well for many different areas where we'd like to know more, or even be able to contribute to changes in a positive way."

FLP is particularly beneficial to those who want to develop creative ideas. Looking into the future can help you to see what really works, and help you avoid spending precious time and effort on bad ideas.

What to expect

You can have a face-to-face session with the FLP practitioner or it is possible to conduct a session via Skype.

At the beginning of the session you will be asked what questions or aspects of your future you would like to discover – for example, areas such as health, family, work, the world, and even your best possible future. Then you will be taken through a gentle meditative journey. You will be asked to visualize a beautiful building, such as a castle. When you climb to the first floor, there will be a corridor lined with doors, each of which relates to one of your questions. As you open the door to each room, you are given an insight into your life five years or so hence.

SELF-HELP

It is easy to do FLP at home using books such as Lorraine Flaherty's *Healing with Past Life Therapy* and Anne Jirsch's *The Future is Yours*, which clearly describe how to do the FLP techniques for many different aspects of the future. Alternatively you can download a future-life progression free from Anne's website (see page 390) or from Lorraine's *Inner Freedom* CD collection, which is also available from Amazon on MP3 for a nominal fee.

Although FLP sessions can be held over Skype, a face-to-face session with a practitioner is more common.

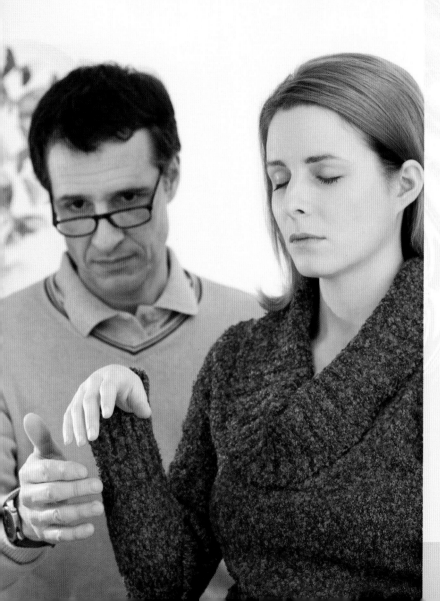

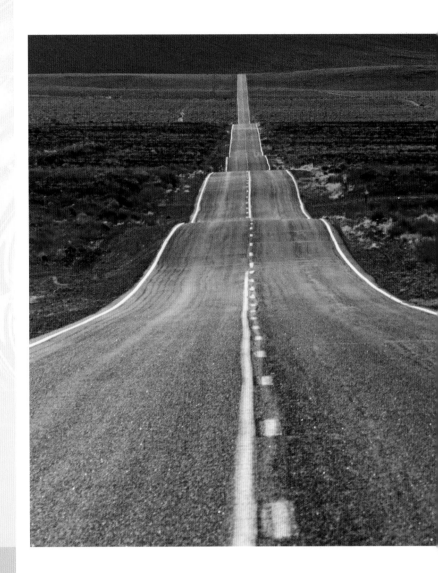

Sometimes you will see nothing in a certain room, which can be disconcerting. However, most practitioners will reassure you that this means there is nothing of great importance or change in that area; instead you can focus on the bigger picture. Hence, nothing to worry about. As you go into other rooms, a clearer scene may present itself, and this information can prove very useful and reassuring when you return from the meditative journey. It

Your future lives can also be accessed using FLP techniques.

STUDY FACT

With FLP it is even possible to access your future lives, going hundreds of years forward into the future, from where you can gain insights and learn from the experiences you will have then. You can also get an overview of our world in the future, and how it and the people within it are changing.

may be something you choose to act upon, or it may just be good to know that things are shaping up okay for you.

All the time the practitioner is prompting you with various questions. Perhaps you want to explore alternative life paths, to see who or what you no longer want in your future life, or what you need to bring in. You may be asked to look at what other opportunities are available to you.

Training

The Past and Future Life Society (see page 390) is the only professional body for past-life regression (see page 296) and future-life progression practitioners. All therapists are fully trained and have reached a high level of competence, adhering to the PFLS code of ethics. They have a list of trained therapists in your area, and also offer training schemes.

Akashic Record therapy

The Akashic Records are believed to be a library – on an energetic or etheric level of existence – which stores records of all you have ever thought, said, and done (or will do), in this life, past lives, future lives, and even in-between lives before your soul reincarnates. Your whole soul's journey is there, from first reincarnation to last.

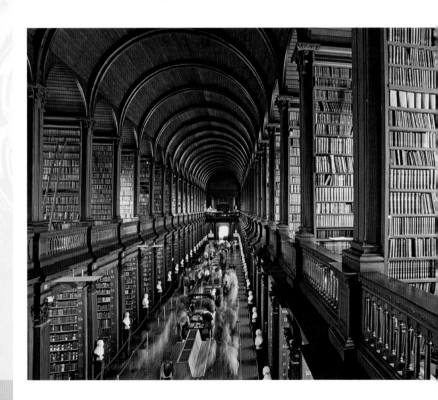

Anyone can tap into this energy database, which is also known as the "universal computer" or "collective unconscious", by doing a specific guided meditation or past-life regression (see page 296), or by allowing an intuitive Akashic Record reader to tune into it remotely and give you a reading of what they discover.

Accessing these etheric Akashic Records brings insight, empowerment, and transformation, helping to clear blockages to happiness, which have usually been repeating over many lives. So instead of feeling held back by obstacles or by making unconscious negative choices, after an Akashic Record healing you will feel free to lead a more purposeful, successful, and fulfilling life.

Amanda Romania, an inspirational life-coach and author of *Akashic Therapy*, explains on her website (see page 390), "In the Akashic Records, each one of us has a divine purpose that is always known to our souls.

The Akashic Records are a store of all past, present, and future life experiences.

It waits to be remembered by us in our human lives. When we awaken to our destiny, we are truly able to self-actualize the imprint of our inspiration for the world to know."

History

The word *akasha* comes from the Sanskrit for sky, space, or ether, and was used by the theosophy pioneer Madame Blavatsky to mean "life force". The Akashic Records are a metaphysical concept, first made popular by theosophists such as Alfred Percy Sinnett, who, in his book *Esoteric Buddhism* (1884), wrote about a Buddhist belief in "a permanency of records in the Akasha", while Charles Webster Leadbeater, in his book *Clairvoyance* (1899), wrote about it as something that a clairvoyant could read.

Another theosophist author Alice Bailey also wrote about the Akashic Record as being like "an immense photographic film, registering all the desires and earth experiences of our planet". She believed that anyone who could perceive it would see "the life experiences of every human being since time began, the reactions to experience of the entire animal kingdom, the aggregation of the thought-forms of a karmic nature (based on desire) of every human unit throughout time". So not only can you see actual events, but also astral pictures created by imagination and desire.

Two of the most famous readers of the Akashic Records were the American psychic Edgar Cayce (1877–1945), and the philosopher, social reformer, and spiritual teacher Rudolf Steiner (1861–1925), who accessed and wrote about the Akashic Records, as well as the evidence he saw of the lost civilizations of Atlantis and Lemuria.

Who can benefit?

Therapy from accessing your Akashic Records can help you understand the root cause, and make lasting change, if you experience constant bad luck, trauma, and negative energies, such as anger, sadness, hatred, or exhaustion. It can shine a light on repeating dramas and difficulties in your relationships, feelings of low confidence, and lack of self-love, and explain why you feel stuck and unfulfilled in life.

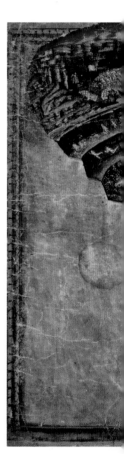

Not only can viewers of the Akashic Records see actual events; they also see astral pictures created by imagination and desire.

If you wonder what your life purpose really is, who you are at a soul level, or if are looking for more spiritual growth, then this therapy will bring clarity, confidence, and the drive to move forward with your life, by giving you a real sense of who

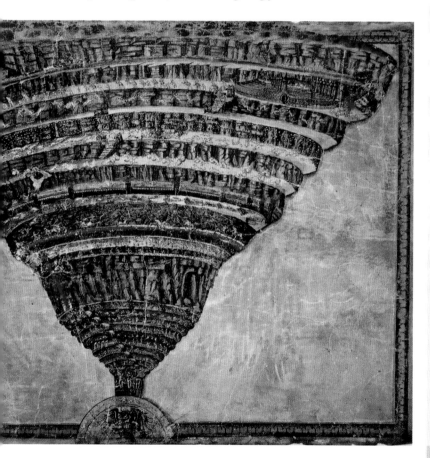

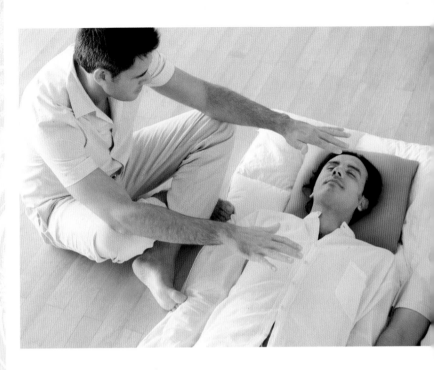

you are and what you are here for. Ultimately it connects you to the Source again, so that you can realize your oneness with the Spirit/Divinity and feel the joy and positivity that come with that.

A practitioner will guide you through a meditation during which you explore records and past or future lives.

What to expect

Healing your Akashic Records yourself, or with a practitioner doing it for you, involves a relaxing session, lying down, fully clothed, and being guided through a meditation in which you get to explore the records, a specific past or future life, or even go to the life between lives, to see what your soul signed up to in this incarnation. A trained practitioner will guide you through a gentle visualization process, where you remain conscious but able to connect with imagery from these various lives, and can recall details when asked specific questions throughout the meditation. This will help you deal with the pain from past lives, learn about your purpose, and heal repeating patterns that may be inhibiting you in this life.

Expect to experience some enlightening realizations; tears and deep emotions may come up, as you go back over events and emotions of a past life that resonates with this present one, or as you become aware of beings from other dimensions, such as the angelic realm, guiding you on your path.

Training

Healer and author Linda Howe has written three books on using the Akashic Records for transforming your life: *How to Read the Akashic Records, Healing Through the Akashic Records,* and *Discover Your Soul's Path Through the Akashic*

Records. In 2001 she set up her own Center for Akashic Studies, "with the intention of using the Akashic Records for personal empowerment, consciousness development, and expanded spiritual awareness". You can find her books, and more details about her one-to-one consultations and coaching, live and online classes, and workshops on her website (see page 390).

At the Soul Realignment website (see page 390) you can sign up and follow a free, three-video course that teaches you how to access and clear your Akashic Records, which is also known as "soul realignment". There is also a Level One training programme – a longer, more in-depth home-study course on which you learn more about soul groups, life purpose, attuning to the Akashic Records, and permanently realigning the negative blocks and influences that you find to bring about great shifts and change in your own or others' lives.

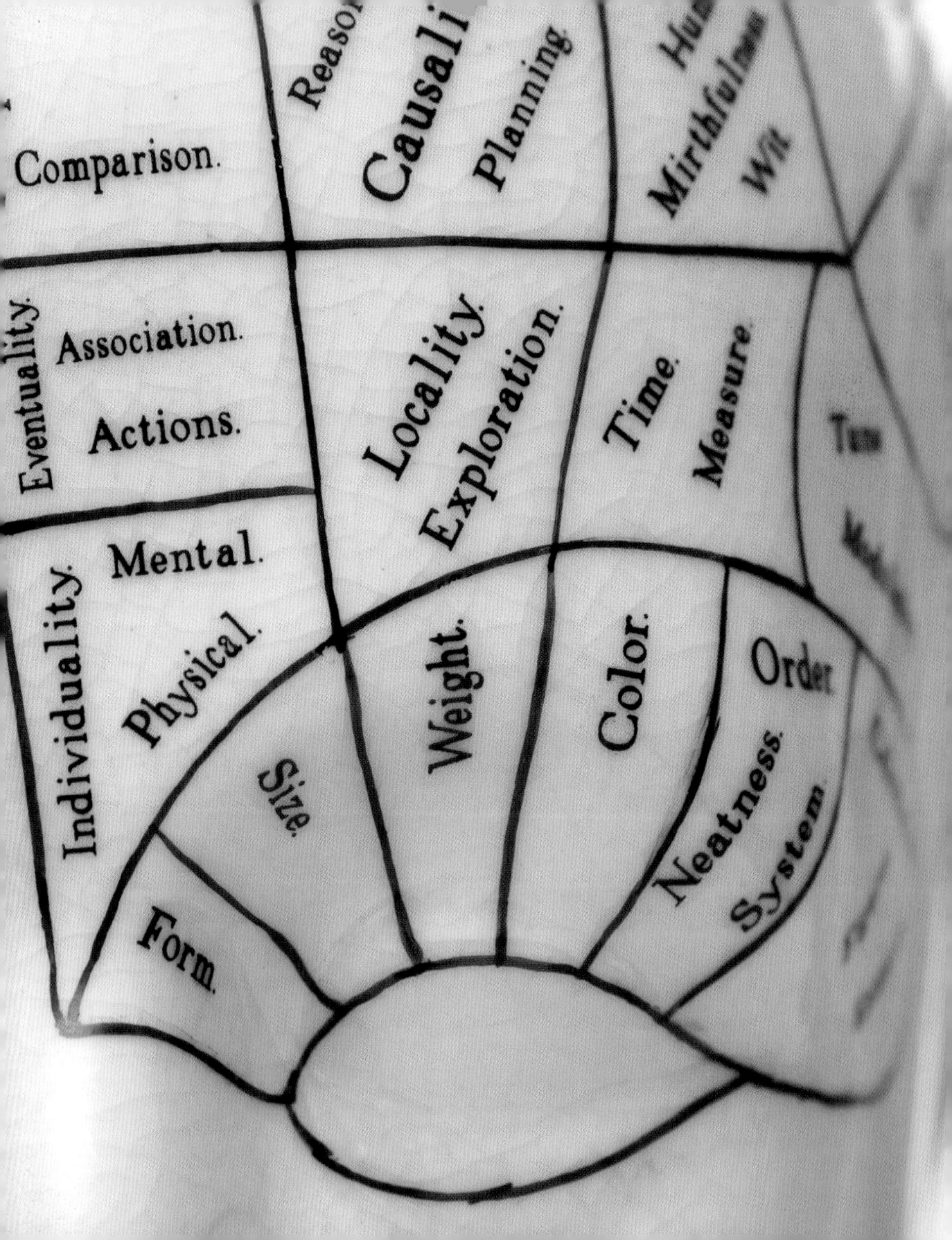

Comparison.

Reason

Causali

Planning

Hu

Mirthfulness

Wit

Eventuality.

Association.

Actions.

Locality.

Exploration.

Time.

Measure.

Ten

Individuality.

Mental.

Physical.

Weight.

Color.

Order

Neatness.

System

Size.

Form.

MIND AND PSYCHOLOGICAL TECHNIQUES

Sophrology

Sophrology? This holistic therapy is widely used and respected throughout continental Europe and America, although the word may not ring many bells in the UK at present. Interest is growing in the benefits that sophrology has to offer to our health and well-being.

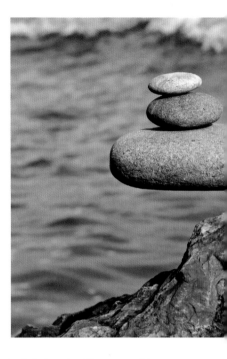

Sophrology means "the science of the consciousness in harmony". It is a life-balancing technique, comprising practical physical and mental exercises aimed at an alert mind in a relaxed body. It is simple and does not require complicated postures or large amounts of time each day. The therapy was created in 1960 in Spain by a neuropsychiatrist, Professor Alfonso Caycedo, who described it as both a philosophy and a way of life, as well as a therapy and a personal development technique. He later added, "sophrology is learning to live."

It is inspired by yoga nidra ("lucid sleeping"), Buddhist meditation, Japanese Zen, and classical relaxation techniques. It has structured sets of exercises that can be done sitting down, lying down, or even standing up. It is not a hands-on therapy; you are guided by the voice of the sophrologist, close your eyes, and follow simple instructions to learn

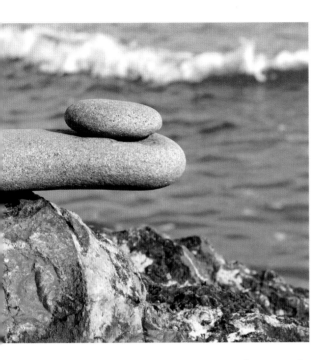

Classical relaxation techniques, such as yoga nidra and meditation, are the inspiration for sophrology.

how to relax, experiment with different breathing techniques, use simple movements, and so on. You can do sophrology on a one-to-one basis or with a group. You learn to quieten the "little voice" in your head, to "switch off" at the end of the day. You do not need to spend a long time each day doing the exercises; they simply fit into your life as it is.

Who can benefit?

Sophrology can be used just as well by the super-busy business person as it can by someone who is lying in bed ill in hospital. The whole idea of sophrology is that anybody can practise this technique, and you do not need to have plenty of spare time on your hands. This therapy can be used for:

- Stress management and anxiety
- Concentration and fatigue
- Insomnia
- Preparation for public speaking, exams, or the stage
- Mental preparation for sports
- Pain management
- Depression
- Birth preparation.

Once you learn the sophrology exercises, they are easy to integrate into your daily life and to practise alone.

What to expect

The idea of sophrology is to be able to stay both calm and alert in the middle of our modern fast-paced, very full life, without having to spend a long time doing postures or meditating while sitting down cross-legged. It is ideal for people who feel they do not have the time to relax.

Sophrology is often thought of as being a relaxation technique,

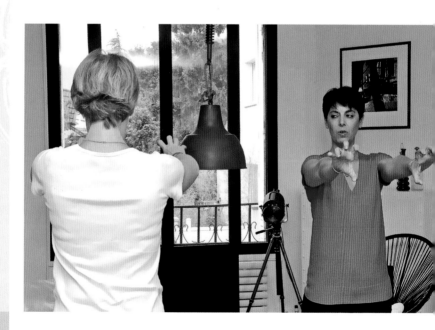

but in fact relaxation is only one of the tools used. Other tools can help you regain energy. So the best word to describe sophrology would probably be "balance", and it can aptly be described as a technique that restores balance in our body, mind, and spirit.

You learn exercises from the sophrologist that you will be able to repeat by yourself on your own: thinking about breathing while you walk or wait for your computer to start; closing your eyes for a few seconds several times a day to regain energy; doing a little "shaking" movement with your shoulders every morning for a couple of minutes, to help manage your stress.

SELF-HELP

Here are a few simple sophrology exercises to try at home:

- **TO LOWER ANXIETY:** Breathe in and gently contract the muscles in your whole body, sensing any tension or discomfort. Breathe out loudly, let go, and completely relax the muscles, letting the tensions flow away. Do this three times, and listen to how you are feeling inside. You can do this exercise sitting down, lying down, or standing up.

- **TO SLEEP BETTER:** Count up to three in your mind as you breathe in, count up to four as you breathe out, and count up to three while you gently hold your breath and your lungs empty; then start all over again. Do this at your own pace, and change the counts if this is better for you, but keep the exercise as regular as you can, until you feel that you are calming down.

- **TO BETTER MANAGE STRESS:** Several times a day, for a few seconds, close your eyes, unclench your jaw, relax your shoulders (let them drop towards the floor), and breathe out loudly.

Meditation

Meditation can take many forms. At its simplest, it means deep contemplation about something. In therapeutic terms, it involves focusing the mind to reach a level of consciousness that is different from that normally experienced, in order to achieve emotional, spiritual, and physical peace and harmony.

Many people derive a wide range of mental benefits from meditation. Relaxation and stress-relief are the major reasons that people turn to it today. Regular meditation can help alleviate hypertension and depression; it can also improve self-confidence for many. Most doctors are only too happy for their patients to use anything that deals successfully with the stresses of modern living, and wholly support making time to relax.

What to expect

Meditation practice varies from teacher to teacher. Most types, such as Tibetan Buddhist meditation, begin with concentrating on breathing; others, including transcendental meditation (TM), use mantras (sounds whose stilling effects have been observed – although you can choose a mantra that is of significance to you).

In yoga the Corpse Pose, or *shavasana*, involves relaxing and meditating while lying flat on your back. Most forms of meditation, however, are carried out in a seated position, so that the spine is straight and the pressures on it are just those of gravity, not of muscular tension. Various techniques are then used to empty the mind of humdrum everyday thoughts: you may begin by counting slowly from one to ten and back down to one again, or by chanting a mantra or picturing a tranquil scene in your mind.

Meditation is used primarily to quieten the mind and to gain insights.

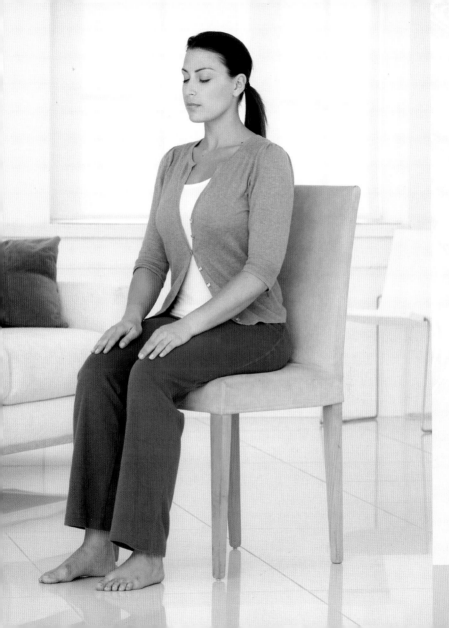

Meditation sessions last for about 30–60 minutes and the costs vary widely, from free community sessions upwards.

The three most commonly recognized forms of meditation are the following:

- **ZEN MEDITATION:** This has long been used by Buddhists for healing in many areas. It involves visualization techniques, and is now used in the West to help heal disease and calm a troubled mind. During deep contemplation, patients are taught to make a mental picture of their disease, and of the effect that treatment has as it works to destroy it.

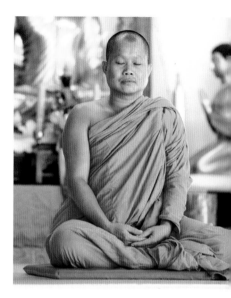

Buddhist meditation is a form of mental concentration that can lead ultimately to enlightenment and spiritual freedom.

- **TRANSCENDENTAL MEDITATION (TM):** This is a popular technique that was developed by friend of the Beatles, the Maharishi Mahesh Yogi (1918–2008). It produces extensively researched benefits to the mind and body through the deep relaxation that is gained. TM is practised silently for 15–20 minutes twice a day, while sitting comfortably with the eyes closed. During the practice the mind settles, and systematically reaches a level of unbounded awareness. At the same time the body's physiology settles to an equally profound level of rest, which TM practitioners believe to be more than twice as deep as that gained during sleep.

- **VIPASSANA MEDITATION:**
  This is one of India's most
  ancient meditation techniques,
  reintroduced for modern
  practice by Ledi Sayadaw
  and Mogok Sayadaw, and
  popularized by S N Goenka.
  It is a non-sectarian technique
  and aims for self-transformation
  through self-observation. By
  paying attention to physical
  sensations in the body (the flow
  of the breath in particular) you
  can develop a healthy mind
  and gain insight into the true
  nature of reality. This is, of
  course, the basis for mindfulness
  practice. A lot of emphasis
  is placed on the heritage of
  Vipassana meditation and the
  preservation of its techniques,
  so teachers do not charge
  for their services (although
  donations are accepted).

Training

Although meditation is widely
practised, there are no governing
organizations for this therapy. You
are best advised to seek personal
recommendations for a teacher,
because learning meditation in a
group can initially be preferable
to self-help. However, once the
technique is perfected, you can
practise meditation on your own,
wherever you find yourself. If you
can't get a good recommendation,
many community groups provide
courses in meditation, and there
are a number of Buddhist and TM
organizations that offer classes.

AUTO-SUGGESTION

Devised by Émile Coué in the
late 19th century, autosuggestion
is based on the belief that the
rapid repetition of mantras – to
reach deeper than the conscious
mind – is helpful in producing
a mind clear of all thoughts and
worries. Coué is the originator
of the famous incantation,
"Every day in every way, I am
getting better and better",
which is used to induce deep
concentration, stimulating the
imagination to believe that the
body and mind can improve.

MINDFULNESS MEDITATION

Mindfulness – a way of paying attention to the present moment and of connecting with ourselves – is known to be successful in helping people with mental and physical health issues, ranging from chronic pain, eating disorders, and addictions to stress, depression, and anxiety. It can also improve your concentration, boost productivity at work, and give you a greater enjoyment of life.

In Western societies we are under greater stress than ever before. Stress is the feeling of being under pressure, with symptoms that include anger and anxiety, difficulty in sleeping, loss of appetite, breathlessness, and chest pain. According to a report by the University of Maryland Medical Center, those who are under prolonged stress are at greater risk of health problems such as high blood pressure and heart attacks.

Mindfulness-based stress reduction (MBSR) incorporates techniques such as meditation, gentle yoga, and mind–body exercises to help you cope with stress. It offers greater clarity about what is happening in your life, improves problem-solving, and boosts concentration.

According to the "Be Mindful" campaign run by the Mental Health Foundation, there is increasing evidence that MBSR can help to reduce anxiety levels and teach new ways to manage stress. The results of clinical studies and research highlight the benefits, such as: a 70 per cent reduction in anxiety; fewer visits to your doctor; longer and better-quality sleep; an increase in disease-fighting antibodies (suggesting improvements to the immune system); a reduction in negative feelings like anger, tension, and depression; and improvements in physical conditions as varied as psoriasis, fibromyalgia, and chronic fatigue syndrome. According to the campaign, the evidence in support of MBSR is so strong that almost 75 per cent of physicians think it would be beneficial for all patients to learn mindfulness-meditation skills, which can be practised anywhere, at any time.

Catherine Kerr, the lead author of a new study into how mindfulness works, says that our attention is "consumed by negative preoccupations, thoughts, and worries" when we are depressed. Rather than extricating ourselves and moving on, we tend to move further into negative thought patterns. Using a "body scanning" technique, mindfulness can help us to control this vicious circle by working through the body, consciously engaging and disengaging with the sensations that are found there. As you do so, alpha rhythms in the brain (organizing the flow of sensory information) increase and decrease. Kerr calls this effect the "sensory volume knob"; it is the ability to focus flexibly, which, the paper proposes, "regulates attention so that it does not become biased toward negative physical sensations and thoughts, as in depression".

Of course this is not new. Some 2,500 years ago early Buddhists expounded a similar theory in the celebrated practice text called *Mindfulness of the Body and Breath*.

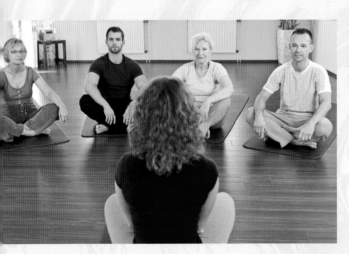

Mindfulness can help you to control negative thought patterns and to alleviate stress.

Psychotherapy

Psychotherapy is one of the talking therapies (others are counselling and psychodynamic therapy). A psychotherapist helps people with emotional, social, or mental-health problems.

During your sessions with a psychotherapist you should feel free to express your feelings. Psychotherapy sessions are confidential, so you can talk about anything that is troubling you or that you cannot talk about with others. Psychotherapy is designed to help you find better ways to cope, or to help you alter the way you think and behave, so that you end up feeling emotionally and mentally stronger.

STUDY FACT

Research suggests that psychological therapies including cognitive behaviour therapy (CBT) – the so-called "talking therapies" – can be beneficial in the treatment of psychotic experiences. In fact, in the UK the National Institute for Health and Care Excellence (NICE) recommends that psychotherapy and CBT should be made available to everyone who is diagnosed with psychosis or schizophrenia.

Who can benefit?

The discipline of psychotherapy comprises a variety of different approaches and methods, ranging from one-to-one talking sessions to therapies involving the use of role-play or dance to explore the emotions. Some therapists specialize in working with couples, families, or groups whose members share similar problems. Psychotherapy is also suitable for adolescents and children.

Psychotherapy is one of the best-known forms of talking therapy.

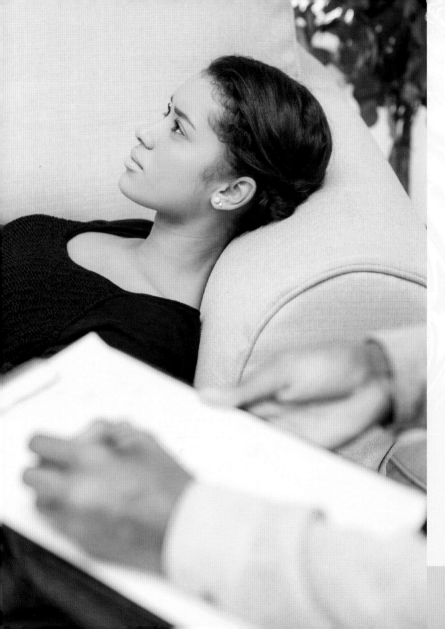

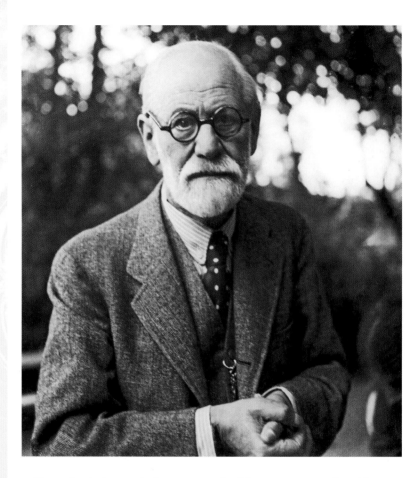

Therapists help people from every background and every part of society. You can access a psychotherapist through your healthcare system or through private practice. Therapists are trained to deal with a diverse range of situations, including:

*Sigmund Freud is the founding father
of psychotherapy.*

- Helping people to deal with
  depression, stress, trauma,
  or phobias
- Assisting children after their
  parents' divorce
- Accelerating recovery from
  brain injury
- Helping people to cope with
  anxiety and bereavement
- Assisting couples who are having
  relationship difficulties
- Aiding personal problem-solving
- Helping those who have
  particular emotional or mental-
  health problems
- Helping a child who has
  problems with academic work
  or behaviour in school, or who
  has suffered bullying or abuse.

What to expect
If you have chosen a therapist
on the basis of personal
recommendation, make sure
you ask them about the process
they are choosing to follow, as
there are many different types
of psychotherapy, including
psychodynamic (psychoanalytic)

PSYCHODYNAMIC PSYCHOTHERAPY

The emphasis in psychodynamic
psychotherapy is on the way
the unconscious and past
experience can influence current
behaviour. You are encouraged
to talk about your childhood
relationships with your parents
and significant others, and the
therapist focuses on how your
client–therapist relationship is
working, often using a method
called "transference" – that is,
the client projects feelings he or
she has experienced in previous
significant relationships onto
the therapist.

The origins of psychodynamics
can be traced right back to
psychoanalysis, although this
approach often offers a quicker
resolution of emotional issues.

GESTALT THERAPY

Gestalt therapy was devised by the German-born psychotherapist Fritz Perls (1893–1970) to focus on a person's experiences, from their feelings and thoughts to their actions. Its name comes from the German word for "organised whole".

It is so easy to get "stuck" in old patterns of behaviour and fixed ideas, and this can block your communication and contact with others. Gestalt therapy puts the emphasis on helping you to develop more awareness of

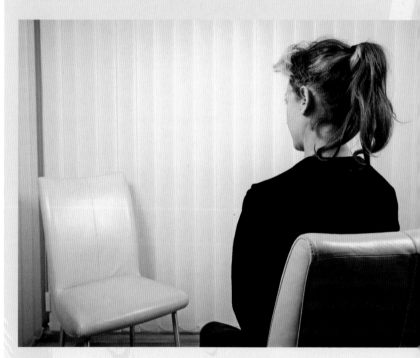

your ideas and behaviours. This is supported by focusing on the "here and now" within the therapy session.

You can gain significant self-awareness by analysing your behaviour and body language, and by expressing your feelings. With this approach you may be invited to "act out" scenarios or to use dream recall. Many Gestalt therapists make use of something called the "open chair" technique. This involves the client sitting opposite an empty chair; they mentally picture sitting in the chair someone who has caused them pain or difficulties. Then they tell the "person" in the empty chair everything they have been unable to express up till now. Sometimes a client is encouraged to swap chairs, in order to reply to the accusations from the perspective of the other person. This is a powerful technique that can give rise to emotional scenes, and the emotions that arise need to be handled with care. So make sure that you consult an experienced, fully qualified Gestalt therapist.

Gestalt therapy is effective with individuals, couples, families, and in groupwork settings. It also offers good results for a wide range of difficulties, and treatment can be either short-term or long-term.

Getstalt therapy helps you to develop greater awareness of your ideas and behaviours.

psychotherapy, cognitive behaviour therapy (CBT), family and marital therapy, cognitive analytical therapy (CAT), interpersonal therapy, dialectic behaviour therapy, and counselling. That way you will know from the outset what to expect.

During the initial assessment or first session, be prepared to trust your instincts, because your relationship with your therapist is central to the process. If you are unsure, seek another therapist. Having confidence in your therapist's abilities is important and will enable you to get the best out of the process.

Whether you need a short- or long-term course of sessions will depend on you (and how complex the issues that you want to resolve might be), your therapist, and the type of therapy. Even so, it is unusual for therapy to take fewer than six sessions, and some types of therapy may last for years. Sessions usually last for 50–60 minutes, depending on your needs – just talk it over with your therapist.

Training

You want to make sure that you are being helped by a therapist who is a member of a suitable professional body in your own country. If you want to ascertain a therapist's qualifications, contact their professional body, which should have the details.

If you wish to train as a psychotherapist, you can apply for a place on an accredited training course with one of the members of your country's professional association. During training you will normally have to undertake in the region of 400–500 hours of college-based therapy training. Within psychotherapy, there are many different modalities, so if you are thinking about training, it is worth researching them all, to see which one appeals the most.

Neuro-linguistic programming

Neuro-linguistic programming (NLP) was created by its co-founders, Richard Bandler and John Grinder, in the 1970s when they embarked on modelling technology work to capture the patterns of genius in Fritz Perls (the developer of Gestalt therapy, see page 332), author and social worker Virginia Satir, and psychiatrist and psychotherapist Milton Erickson. The therapy explores how we think (*neuro*), how we speak (*linguistic*), and how we act (*programming*) – and, ultimately, how all three interact to have a positive (or negative) effect on each of us.

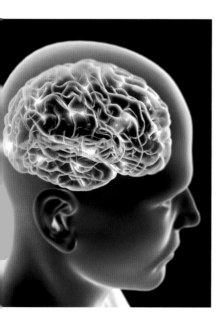

STUDY FACT

Do not confuse NLP with neuro-linguistic psychotherapy, which is a different discipline. In Britain therapists specializing in neuro-linguistic psychotherapy are registered with the UK Council for Psychotherapy and are required to have undergone a minimum of four years' clinical training.

The interaction of how we think, speak, and act has a profound effect upon each of us.

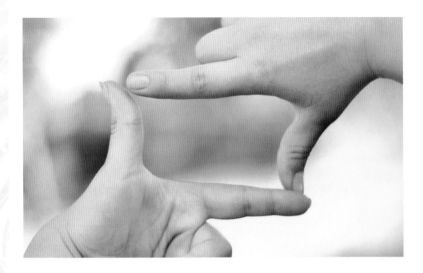

Using a wide range of methods and models, NLP helps you to understand your thought processes and behaviour so that you can make positive changes. As an NLP student, you gain insights into how your thought patterns can affect every facet of your life.

A key element of NLP is that we form unique internal mental maps of the world, as a product of the way we filter and perceive information that is absorbed through our five senses from the world around us. NLP is the study of how a combination

NLP gives you an insight into how your thought patterns affect every facet of your life.

of conscious and unconscious processes enables people to act as they do. Often the answers are not known at a conscious level, but, using NLP, we can extract the unfamiliar pieces.

Whether you want to improve your relationships, remove anxiety, or compete more effectively in the marketplace, the keys to the puzzle can be found in your inner thoughts – in the form of words, images, feelings, or even beliefs. As you discover the unknown pieces, so you can change them, if you want to. You can liken NLP exercises to psychological games or mental exercises.

Who can benefit?

NLP can bring about long-lasting results extremely quickly, and it can be used effectively for both individuals and organizations. It can be beneficial not only in helping overcome issues such as anxiety and stress, lack of confidence, dyslexia, and fears and phobias, but also in enhancing skills and performance in areas such as business, arts and creativity, education, presentation, sport, relationships, and parenting.

What to expect

You can have one-to-one support, to achieve a specific goal or deal with a particular challenge in your life, by visiting an NLP professional (a practitioner or master practitioner). In contrast to some other forms of therapy, with NLP you do not have to reveal any painful secrets – only those which you are happy to disclose.

A short period of time is spent on defining the problem, before work commences on the outcomes, so you should see change in each session. Most people will need only around one to three two-hour sessions of NLP. The sessions are friendly and relaxed, and should not be gruelling in any way.

Training

If you would like to learn more about NLP, either for your own personal development or because you are considering a career change or additional career, you can attend some NLP training and become a qualified practitioner yourself.

Some training companies focus on the business application of NLP, while others focus on therapy, so depending on what you want to do, check this out before you commit to a training course. The Association for NLP (ANLP) recommends that you always ask for at least three referees (former students who have undergone the course), to whom you can speak about their experience. Remember that people who do NLP well model the excellence they promote; they are walking, living, talking examples of the potential of this therapy. They are great communicators, and you should feel great around them.

ENERGETIC NLP™

Art Giser founded Energetic NLP™ in 1985, after studying with the founders of NLP and prominent spiritual teachers. This therapy is a toolbox of simple techniques that help you to develop your energy, to allow personal development at every level. You can also use the tools to do energetic healings for others.

Energetic NLP™ draws on and combines the best elements of NLP, transformational energetic work, energy healing, and intuition development. One of its fundamental goals is to bring the eight agendas that rule your life (and which are often in conflict with each other) into a collaborative relationship with one another. The eight agendas are:

• Your conscious mind's agenda
• The separate agendas of each part of your unconscious mind
• Your soul's agenda
• Your spirit's agenda
• Your physical body's agenda
• The agenda of groups that you are connected to (nationalities, religions, families, and so on)
• Humanity's collective agenda
• And, depending on your beliefs, you may wish to add another category of agendas: God's, the Great Spirit's, or the universe's.

Emotional freedom techniques/tapping

Emotional freedom techniques (EFT), or tapping, is literally a hands-on approach to problem-solving, clearing the energy blocks in the mind–body system that may be interrupting your healing processes.

EFT works by clearing the blockage or disruption by tapping on the endpoints of the body's energy meridians (while thinking of a specific issue), which sends pulses of energy to rebalance the body's energy system in relation to that thought or specific issue. Shifting the energy changes the way the brain processes information about a particular issue. And so tapping, while tuned into an issue, is like rewiring or rerouting the brain's conditioned negative response.

You can imagine how liberating this is if you, or someone you know, has suffered from a phobia or traumatic memories. EFT also works in the same way to release the limiting thoughts and beliefs that get in the way of success, happiness, health, and inner peace.

History

Developed by Gary Craig in the US in the 1990s, EFT is one of the leading techniques of the new-generation treatments that are referred to as "energy psychology". The success of these treatments with a wide range of emotional and physical issues is creating breakthrough understandings about the nature of healing and personal change.

Who can benefit?

EFT is often used as a treatment tool for those suffering from anxieties, fears, trauma, procrastination, addictions, weight loss, and much more. It is a gentle way to transform any issues that are blocking emotional happiness or personal achievement. Other conditions

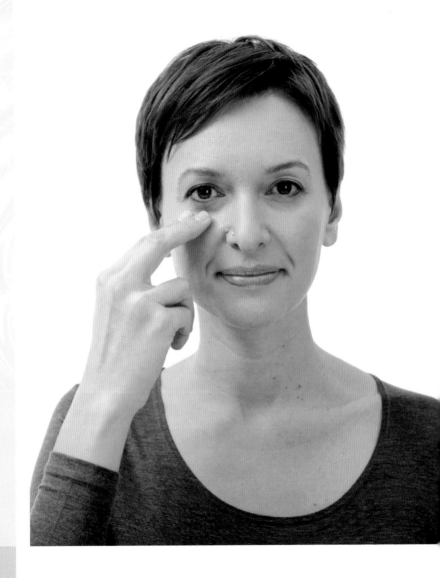

that are listed as suitable for treatment include:

- Pain relief
- Eating disorders
- Post-traumatic stress disorder (PTSD)
- Abuse
- Depression
- Dyslexia
- Attention deficit (hyperactivity) disorder (ADD/ADHD)
- Diabetes
- Allergies
- Obsessive-compulsive disorder (OCD)
- Carpal tunnel syndrome
- Blood-pressure issues
- Headaches.

What to expect

EFT is a powerful self-help tool, as well as a treatment that can be given by a trained practitioner.

In the Set Up stage, you begin with an affirmation (a positive assertion) that is repeated three times, while tapping the side

Tapping a specific point while repeating an affirmation is a powerful way in which to reprogramme subconscious negative thoughts.

of your hand (the karate-chop point). The affirmation is used to correct psychological reversal (PR), which is the energetic equivalent of self-sabotage and is caused by subconscious negative thought patterns and limiting beliefs. So, for example, your affirmation might be, "Even though **I feel sad**, I deeply and completely accept myself." The phrase in bold is the reminder phrase, which you then repeat as you tap various points on the body, to remind your unconscious mind what you are working on. The affirmation and the reminder phase are adjusted as the issues reduce.

Unlike acupuncture, where the practitioner needs to be very

STUDY FACT

EFT is one modality within the "integrated energy techniques" and complements other modalities within the field, as well as being compatible with other therapies.

precise when positioning their needles, with EFT there is more flexibility. As long as you are tapping in the right general area, you do not need to worry about being exactly on the point, as the meridians flow all over the body.

Using a practitioner

Why go to a practitioner, when EFT is such an effective self-help tool? Indeed, it is possible to get extraordinary change with even the most basic knowledge of EFT, using self-help and little or no

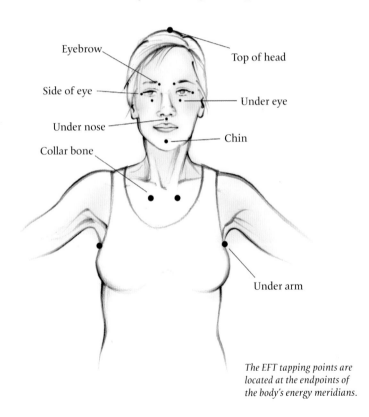

Eyebrow

Top of head

Side of eye

Under eye

Under nose

Chin

Collar bone

Under arm

The EFT tapping points are located at the endpoints of the body's energy meridians.

understanding of the "science" and thinking behind it. However, there are times when EFT doesn't seem to work through self-help.

This is when the practitioner comes in – when you are stuck. Their role is to be there when self-tapping comes up against a block; to be the detective, and to use language skills to creatively assist you to unearth your core issues and beliefs; to question them in ways that you wouldn't think of doing yourself. Often the creative language and questioning skills of the practitioner are invaluable in allowing the process to flow smoothly. The marriage of EFT and NLP (see page 335) is a powerful and effective union.

The role of the practitioner is also to keep the client focused (to be a kind but firm guide to your process), and to gently help you resolve your issues in a supportive and comfortable environment; to keep you not just on track, but moving forward.

The number of sessions required will depend on the complexity of the issue, and it is important to bear in mind that while some problems (or parts of a problem) will clear straight away, there may be deeper aspects involved, which will require time, patience, and the expert skill of an experienced, creative practitioner to achieve a complete result.

One of the great benefits of EFT is that complex work can take place either face-to-face or on the telephone.

Training

There are 29 EFT founding masters worldwide – experienced professional therapists, trainers, and coaches who put EFT at the centre of their practice. All have been developing their skills for many years and have passed a rigorous practical and written examination with EFT founder Gary Craig. You can learn from the masters through their trainings, workshops, retreats, group and individual work; or you can read their books and articles.

Picture-tapping technique

Did you know that if you have an issue you want to deal with, but are not comfortable vocalizing the details, you can obtain dramatic and permanent shifts away from the negative emotion through the picture-tapping technique (PTT)? This is an energy psychology technique developed by Philip Davis and Christine Sutton in 2009, which uses the basics of EFT (see page 339) – that is, tapping on the meridian points – along with the power of the metaphor and the imagination. Using this combination, you can release problems without pain.

For clients who feel they cannot talk (or are uncomfortable with talking) about an issue, this therapy allows them to receive the benefits of EFT by expressing their feelings through drawing. PTT gives them an insight into facets, thoughts, and memories

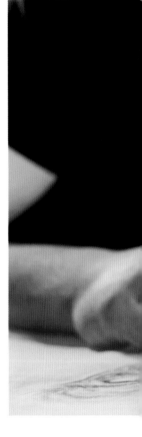

Picture-tapping technique is drawn from EFT and is ideal for clients who feel uncomfortable or unable to talk about an issue.

that may be difficult to express verbally or using other therapies. Clients are frequently amazed, and relieved, at the way things are resolved, and at the connections

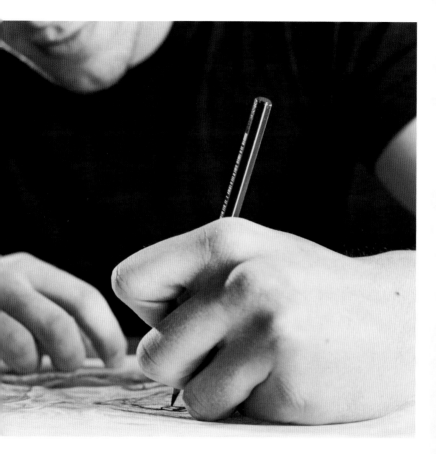

between events and issues that are brought to light.

Many people say they cannot draw, but that is not a problem, for PTT is not an artistic exercise, but a chance to allow your subconscious to manifest itself through visual imagery. The subconscious is where all issues are stored and where the healing takes place.

Who can benefit?

Everybody can put pen to paper to create an image, and so everyone can avail themselves of this technique. It can be used to bring about resolution for people who are experiencing stress around issues that are unspecific, such as low self-esteem, depression, or anxiety.

Some of the areas to which PTT can be applied are as follows:

- Lack of self-confidence
- Low self-esteem
- Job/work issues
- Family issues
- Partner relationships
- Financial worries
- Blocks to success
- Karma from past lives
- Writer's block
- Fear of the new
- Health concerns.

What to expect

The therapist asks the client to connect with the issue they wish to resolve. They can draw their issue in any way they choose, as it is *their* problem and *their* mind that will portray the issue.

So, handing them a blank sheet of paper, the therapist asks the client to draw the issue as it feels to them. After a minute or two the therapist will ask if the picture is complete, and whether the client is satisfied that it portrays the issue. If so, the client will be asked if they would like to assign a title to it.

At this stage the therapist will direct the client to follow them in tapping on the EFT points (as in traditional EFT routines), and will simultaneously ask the client to describe their picture factually and in detail. What is needed here is a description of what they drew, what colours they used, and where on the page the components are. The therapist may intervene and ask for clarification, such as what shade of red the client had chosen.

The client is then asked if they feel resolution has been achieved; if not, another round of drawing and tapping follows. In fact several rounds of drawings are often required before the client feels that a resolution has been arrived at, and the final picture will represent this resolution.

At each round of drawing and tapping there will be a noticeable shift away from the negative emotions associated with the problem, towards a more stable and positive state in the client. Each time the therapist will check in with the client to assess where they are in reaching that resolution in their mind.

Once resolution has been achieved, the client will be asked to visualize putting a frame around the resolution picture. They are asked to describe this frame, and are then asked to make it brighter and bigger, and for all the colours of the resolution

Tapping on EFT points is still a part of PTT.

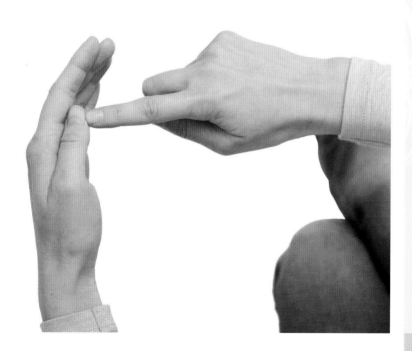

image to be treated similarly. This is the positive image that the client requires, so they are then invited to visualize this bright colour (or colour combination) over their heads, and then making its way down through every part of their being, right down to cellular level, where the positive image is imprinted. Particular attention is given to areas where they may have been feeling pain associated with the issue, so that this imprinting of the positive energy can be directed more in those places.

The effectiveness of the therapy session is tested by the client being asked to view all of the pictures in sequence, laid out in front of them, in the order in which they were drawn; and then asked to assess if there is any emotional reaction to them. It is usual that at this stage the emotions have been moved to positive, happier feelings. However, any negative emotions would indicate that another aspect of the issue has arisen, and that can be managed equally, using the same process. This therapy is so effective and engaging, and at the end the client is in a better place, and the therapist did not even need to know what the actual issue was.

PTT FOR CHILDREN

This technique works wonderfully with children too, because drawing is something they enjoy doing, and it means they don't have to verbalize their problems. In fact, with a crayon in hand, children are often far less inhibited in expressing themselves, compared to adults! Because the problem is expressed metaphorically – in the image that is drawn – the problem of not being able to express the issue verbally is easily overcome.

Matrix reimprinting

Matrix reimprinting (MR) is a relatively new branch of energy psychology, or meridian-tapping therapy, that was created by EFT master Karl Dawson. It evolved from the popular self-help therapy of emotional freedom techniques (EFT, see page 339) and is known for its ability to quickly transform your relationship to your past, creating shifts in your emotional and physical well-being in the present moment. Through the application of MR you can be free of the pain of past traumas and thus transform your life.

MR is increasingly popular because of its gentleness and effectiveness in the management of emotional or physical issues. It incorporates elements of EFT, NLP (see page 335), regression hypnosis, and quantum physics, and also acknowledges the meridian system of Traditional Chinese Medicine (see page 80).

One key point in MR is that at the time of traumatic events in your past (especially your younger years) you formed certain beliefs that you carry with you to the present, and these affect your physical and mental well-being. Conventional EFT removes the emotional intensity from a past memory, so that you are able to recall the most traumatic and stressful life memories without any emotional disruption or stress. However, matrix reimprinting allows you to actually revisit a past traumatic event and change that memory – *for ever* – so that you are liberated from the negative emotions and limiting beliefs that you formed at the time of the trauma.

Holding on to traumatic memories of past events can keep the body in a heightened state of stress, which in turn leads to "dis-ease". From a psychological perspective, traumatic memories are frozen in time, and you can become stuck in an endless loop, playing the emotionally upsetting scene over and over again. You then tune into them at a subconscious level, resulting in the trauma affecting your health, your well-being, and your point of attraction.

In matrix reimprinting these frozen memories are referred to as the "ECHOs" – the Energy Consciousness Holograms – of your younger self, your inner child, and so on. It is the ECHO that is the client in this technique. When you revisit a painful traumatic memory in a MR session, you are stepping into

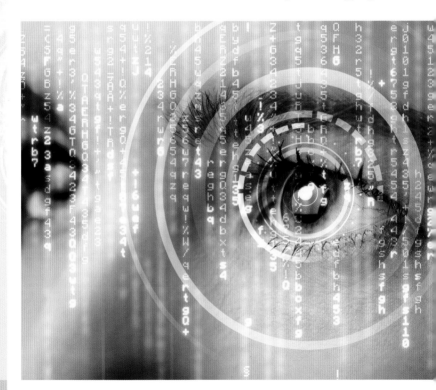

that scene in the matrix and, in a gentle and controlled way, you interact with your ECHOs. In this way you can release the ECHO from the freeze-response and generate a new understanding and resolution to the painful event, reimprinting it with positive beliefs and emotions in your current life.

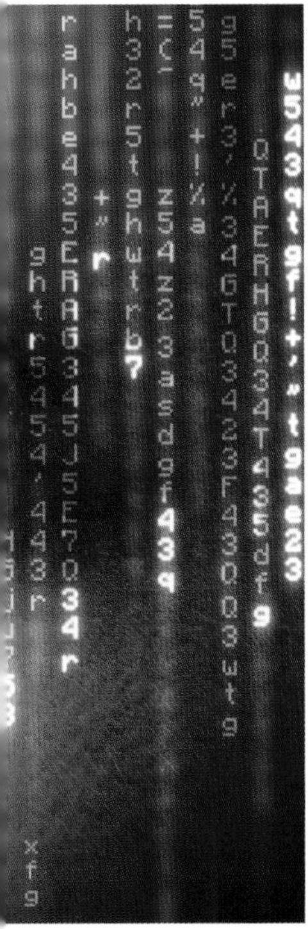

Who can benefit?

Matrix reimprinting has given rise to a whole range of healing protocols, which can transform a wide range of experiences where there was an element of shock or trauma, such as:

- Abuse
- Addictions
- Allergies
- Birth traumas
- Negative core-beliefs
- Phobias
- Relationships
- Sports performance
- Stage/public performance
- Chronic pain
- Chronic illness
- Accidents.

During a matrix reimprinting session, you may step into a painful or traumatic memory in the matrix, but in a controlled and gentle way.

STUDY FACT

Using MR you can even work with past lives and future selves, and enhance your work with the Law of Attraction (see page 369).

As a therapist's tool, MR is excellent in conjunction with life-coaching, counselling, hypnotherapy, psychotherapy, and so on. Regardless of whether it is used alone or with whatever your principal modality is, the inclusion of MR will enable you to generate rapid transformations of life-traumas in your clients or yourself. This in turn returns the body from a heightened state of stress to balance, so that healing can resume.

What to expect

In an MR session you bring to mind, and state, the issue that you want to work with. The practitioner will invite you to step into that scene in your mind, all the while tapping on a particular set of acupuncture points. Tapping on the EFT points accelerates the process. You *interact* with the ECHO (the self in the past event) by reassuring it that you are there to help, empower, and assist the ECHO to obtain release from pain. While revisiting the memory in the matrix, through the ECHO, you can state (and action) what you would have preferred to happen at the time of the specific traumatic event. You can thus bring in new resources to the scene, to create and transform the emotional loading of the events of that memory.

In this way the scene or memory of this event is being changed, with alternative scenarios and feelings. In MR you are not denying or changing historical events, but you are altering the emotional charge and understanding of these events. This process brings about a release from the negative emotions, and replaces these with positive outcomes or new, empowering understanding. In this technique your pain is not retriggered by the events of the painful memory.

Anyone can learn the technique of matrix reimprinting and proceed to work on themselves.

Compassion-focused therapy

Compassion-focused therapy (CFT) was developed to help those who have troubled, neglectful, abusive, or emotionally insecure backgrounds. However, it is also being used to help others who simply need, or want, to develop greater compassion and kindness for themselves and others. It is also showing good results in helping people with a range of difficulties, such as PTSD and personality and eating disorders.

HEALER PROFILE

Paul Gilbert, who is Professor of Clinical Psychology at the University of Derby and a Fellow of the British Psychological Society, is the founder of CFT. He has been working with, and researching, shame-related processes for 30 years, with the emphasis in the past 15 years on looking at compassion as an antidote to shame and self-criticism.

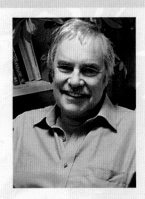

Professor Paul Gilbert is the founder of compassion-focused therapy.

CFT is a result of Professor Gilbert's observations that people often understand that there is no logical reason to feel the way they do, but that doesn't stop them experiencing these emotions. This is where logic and emotion are in conflict – and CFT can help to combat this.

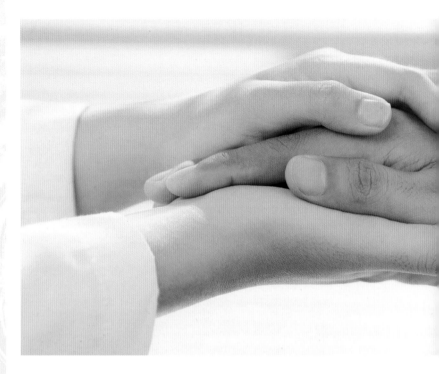

A CFT therapist uses compassion to create feelings of warmth, kindness, and support.

CFT draws on modern neuroscience, cognitive behavioural therapies (CBT), and traditional Buddhist practices, and can best be described as an "integrated and multimodal approach". The practitioner works closely with the client to help identify their behavioural and emotional responses, and to find ways to rebalance these, so that not only does the client feel better, but is better able to show the qualities of compassion, kindness, and sympathy to others as well as themselves.

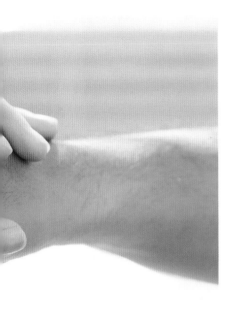

- The contentment-, soothing- and affiliative-focused system.

Although all three systems have been shown to have important effects on other abilities, such as our capacity for attention, tolerating distress, and mentalizing (being able to understand the mental states that underlie behaviour), it is well recognized that kindness and support for oneself (or from others) can help to soothe threats and restore a sense of safeness. Mindful compassion enables us to hold these three systems in mind, and creates a sense of choice around which one we cultivate.

Using the "it's-not-our-fault" approach, a lot of time is spent on normalizing and de-shaming emotional responses, and on understanding the distinction between taking responsibility for them and condemning and blaming behaviours. There is a good deal of time spent in discussion, with a calming and soothing orientation that "we are all in this together".

Emotion-regulation systems

Fundamentally, research shows that we have at least three types of emotion-regulation systems:

- The threat-detection and protection-focused system
- The drive- and excitement- focused system

Who can benefit?

CFT was originally developed for those who experience high levels of shame and self-criticism – often people with complex mental-health difficulties who come from neglectful backgrounds. However, in recent years CFT has been found to offer good results for people suffering with depression and anxiety, too.

Eating disorders is another area where CFT is developing distinctly and getting good outcomes. And it is starting to be used in relationship counselling too, to help couples understand each other's threat systems.

Throughout the process the therapist will use compassion to create feelings of warmth, kindness, and support and will be sensitive to whether or not the patient is trying to force (or even bully) themselves to change, rather than being supportive and encouraging in their efforts.

What to expect

Initially the therapist is likely to use the "three-circle model" – asking the client to draw circles with pen and paper, to show how much they feel the "threat", "drive", and "soothing" systems (see page 355). Working together, the therapist and individual will then make sense of their experiences, including the ways in which they have coped and the unintended consequences these can bring. Together they will then work out what might be helpful for the individual.

The next step is to use compassionate mind training (see the box opposite) to develop a "compassionate self".

STUDY FACT

Professor Gilbert's latest research focus is on the fear of positive emotion: exploring how many people fear that if they are happy today, "something bad will happen tomorrow", plus the fear of compassion and/ or myths about compassion (such as loving oneself).

Training

For psychotherapists and counsellors who wish to train in CFT, there are introductory and more advanced workshops available in the UK through the Compassionate Mind Foundation (see page 391). For those in other countries, check on the Internet for similar associations and organizations that offer advice and training.

COMPASSIONATE MIND TRAINING

CFT is the overarching therapy, while "compassionate mind training" (CMT) refers to the exercises and practices in CFT, which can be used by anyone wanting to develop their compassion. For example, you might be invited to imagine compassion flowing out from you to others, and compassion flowing back to you from others (and from yourself). You could be asked to use exercises similar to those used in cognitive behaviour therapy (CBT, see page 363), such as letter-writing, mindfulness, writing dialogues and rescripting them, graded tasks, and chair-work – all with the emphasis on making sure that you feel supported and encouraged.

Obviously the range of exercises is tailored closely to your specific needs and your way of thinking. Although the profound emotional shifts that many experience from practising them, and from showing self-compassion (perhaps for the first time), can be disconcerting or scary, the vast majority of people report feeling enormous benefit from sticking with CFT, and thus being able to connect emotionally and reduce feelings of self-criticism and shame.

F**k It therapy

According to Fk It therapy co-founder, John C Parkin, saying "F**k It" is the perfect way to discover freedom, because you "stop worrying (generally), give up wanting (mainly), and end up being darn happy to be yourself in the present moment (if you're lucky)".**

HEALER PROFILE

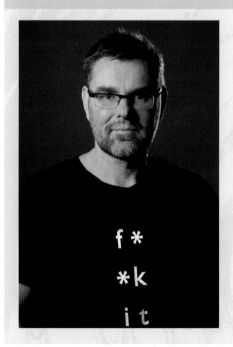

It all sounds a bit too good to be true, but as soon as **John C Parkin** started saying "F**k It", he left the London rat-race and started a new life in the Italian region of Le Marche. Together with his wife, Gaia Pollini, he now runs retreats in Italy, is a bestselling author, and has discovered the freedom to do more of what he wants to do, and less of what people say he should be doing.

*John Parkin is the founder of F**k It Therapy, which he teaches with his wife Gaia Pollini.*

So how can the rest of us start living the F**k It way? Well, you can go on a week-long retreat in one of a number of Italian locations; you can attend a UK/Ireland weekend workshop; you can subscribe to the e-courses; or you can buy one of the F**k It books and manuals.

Who can benefit?

Anyone who questions their current lifestyle or life-purpose, who is uptight and over-stressed, or who seeks a more enlightened way to live could benefit from a F**k It course. For traditionalists who like their spiritual retreats to be structured, reverential, and guru-led, a F**k It week might at first glance appear spiritually "lite". But, despite the laughter and apparent glibness, a very real spiritual process takes place, for the majority of participants. However, if you are the kind of person who likes to follow 12 steps in order to achieve a goal, this may not be the retreat for you, as there is no right or wrong answer or reaction – a point that is heavily stressed throughout the week.

What to expect

The pace of the retreat is slow and relaxed. After a leisurely breakfast, each morning session starts with some gentle qigong practice (see page 125). There are morning (10am–12pm) and afternoon (5pm–7pm) sessions full of interesting, sometimes intense, usually fun tutored exercises, talks, and discussions. Usually some energy work is involved at some point during the week, and often a breathwork session.

After each tutored session, participants are helped to ground themselves by tucking into delicious vegetarian meals. The fresh, organic food is locally sourced and plentiful. Regional Italian wine also flows freely in the evenings, for those who like to wash down their pasta with something more potent than elderflower cordial (which is also available). This retreat is certainly not for those who favour the hair-shirt and abstinence approach.

There is a good deal of time out built into each day, so that you can relax in whatever way suits your mood.

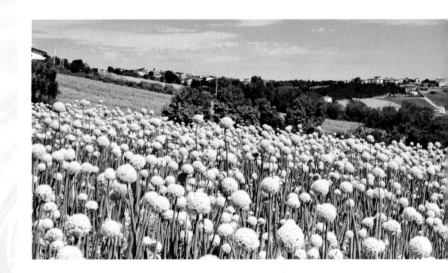

THE AUTHOR'S EXPERIENCE OF A F**K IT RETREAT

As in Taoism, giving up on striving and tension – effectively, taking your hands off the steering wheel and seeing where life leads you – is one of the central tenets of the F**k It retreat. The week-long course is facilitated by John and Gaia, both of whom have spent more than 20 years studying meditation, shamanism, breathwork, and the Eastern philosophies. It was as a result of their spiritual questioning that they came to the conclusion that the process of simplification – neatly summed up by the profanity "F**k It" – could be a profound spiritual process in itself. Once you realize things don't matter as much as you think they do, life starts to get interesting (in Buddhist terms, this is releasing our "attachments").

Initially this is quite a nebulous concept to grasp, but the retreat is well structured, with teaching elements, group exercises, and "sharing" sessions

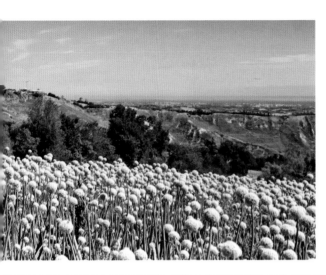

*Letting go of being in control and worrying is all part of a week-long F**k It retreat.*

interspersed with plenty of relaxation, so that eventually these hazy ideas become clearer. As the week progresses, you slowly realize the wisdom of stopping doing what you don't want to, and tuning in to what you *do* really want to do. The problem is that letting go of the things that matter to us (like doing well in our careers, being a good wife/husband/mother/father, or finding our purpose) is something that seems hard to relinquish. However, as we learned from John and Gaia, it shouldn't involve too much effort.

Our breathwork session took place on the penultimate day, leaving some shaken, others elated, and everyone moved. Gaia led the group with focused breathing techniques to get the energy flowing, and to help take us into a state of Oneness. It was a powerful spiritual practice for the vast majority of the group.

GAIA'S MAGIC

Many people came out of a session talking about Gaia's magic. It's hard to put your finger on it exactly, but what she does is just "magic". And, in response to demand, she now runs F**k It Magic weekends and weeks.

Gaia is a powerful breathworker, an expert in *qi* (energy) and qigong, a master of Chinese teas and the tea ceremony, and an experienced and intuitive therapist. She has an uncanny knack of knowing what is going on in people, and is able to give you a blast of energy in just the right place, talk about just the right thing, and create just the right space for you at that particular time.

Although each of Gaia's F**k It Magic weekends is different, the elements of energy work, breathwork, and qigong will always be present.

Gaia performs tea ceremonies as part of her "magic" experience.

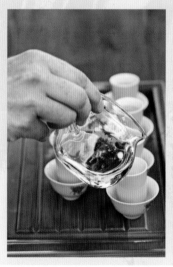
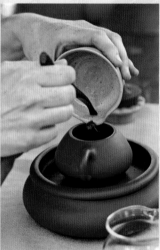

Cognitive behaviour therapy

Cognitive behaviour therapy (CBT) used to be known simply as "cognitive therapy", but because it is almost always practised with behavioural therapy principles, it has become widely known as CBT.

The principles behind it are that if we learn about how our thoughts create our moods, then we can counteract the negative thoughts that tend to make us unhappy or disturbed as they arise, challenge them, and rethink them. CBT helps us to recognize the particular triggers and specific situations that bring about our own specific, inherent tendency to negative thoughts, whatever those might be – such as "I'm unlovable", "I'm not good enough", or "I'm not bright enough". Cognitive therapy teaches us to stop thinking such negative thoughts, and to challenge untrue thoughts and replace them with more rational and healthy ones that are based in reality.

Who can benefit?

There has been a great deal of research into the benefits of cognitive behaviour therapy, which suits individuals with all sorts of problems, including:

- Depression
- Stress and anxiety
- Phobias
- Difficult relationships
- OCD
- Eating disorders, especially anorexia and bulimia nervosa.

Research shows that for some people CBT is more effective than other kinds of treatment, including the use of antidepressants.

What to expect

CBT may be done one-on-one, in groups with family members, or with other people who have similar issues.

At your first session, your therapist will typically gather

information about you and determine what concerns you would like to work on. He or she will probably ask you about your current and past physical and emotional health, in order to gain a deeper understanding of your situation. If you don't feel comfortable with the first therapist you consult, try someone else. Having a good "fit" with your therapist can assist you in getting the most benefit from cognitive behaviour therapy.

HEALER PROFILE

The medical doctor, psychiatrist, and psychoanalyst **Aaron Beck** developed cognitive therapy in the early 1960s while he was a professor at the University of Pennsylvania. Through his work with depressed patients, he noticed that they experienced a flow of negative thoughts that seemed to arise spontaneously. He called these cognitions "automatic thoughts" and realized that their content fell into three categories: negative ideas about themselves, the world, and the future. Patients did not have to spend much time at all reflecting on automatic thoughts before they started to treat them as valid.

Beck began to help his patients to recognize these thoughts and evaluate them. In so doing, patients were able to think more realistically, which in turn helped them to feel better emotionally and to function better. By educating someone to understand and become aware of their distorted thinking, you can challenge its effects.

Beck is the founder and President Emeritus of the not-for-profit Beck Institute for Cognitive Behavior Therapy, which is based in Pennsylvania.

During successive CBT sessions, your therapist will encourage you to talk about your thoughts and feelings and whatever is troubling you. Don't worry if you find it hard to open up about your feelings. Your therapist can help you gain more confidence and comfort.

CBT generally focuses on specific problems, using a goal-oriented approach. You may be asked to do "homework" as you progress – activities, reading, or practices that build on what you learn during your regular therapy sessions – and to apply in your daily life what you are learning.

STUDY FACT

Unlike many other types of psychotherapy (see page 328), CBT is ideally suited to a self-help approach and can be learned through many books, CDs, and online resources (see right).

Typical steps you may go through include:

- Identifying troubling situations or conditions in your life
- Becoming aware of your thoughts, emotions, and beliefs about these situations or conditions; and identifying negative or inaccurate thinking
- Challenging negative or inaccurate thinking.

CBT is generally considered a short-term therapy of about 10–20 sessions.

Training

There are plenty of CBT therapists operating in the private sector, but increasingly in recent years CBT is being offered as part of public health services, because it is being recognized as one of the preferred methods of treatment for mild to moderate depression. So research the situation in your own country.

Self-help CBT media, such as books, CD-ROMS, and online resources (see page 391), are also available. View the websites Beating the Blues for mild to moderate

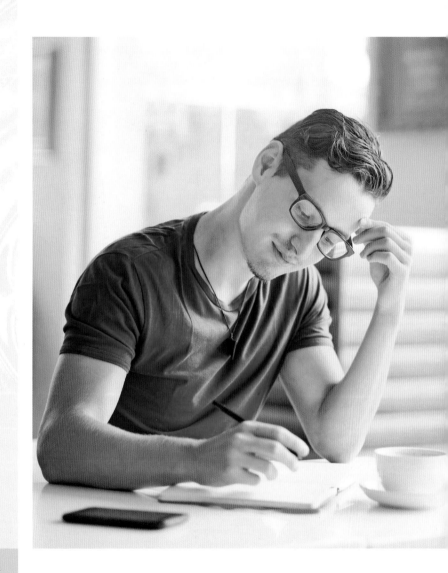

depression and FearFighter for the management of panic and phobia (see page 391). Ask at your doctor's practice if you would like to do this under their supervision.

Exercises to build on what you learn during your CBT sessions are all part of this "goal-oriented" approach.

There is also a free online service set up by the psychiatrist Dr Chris Williams, which anyone anywhere can access – you simply have to register. The website is called Living Life to the Full (see page 391).

RATIONAL EMOTIVE BEHAVIOUR THERAPY

At much the same time as Aaron Beck was formulating his ideas on CBT, another therapist, Albert Ellis (1913–2007), was coming to much the same conclusions about patients' negative thoughts and their tendencies to "catastrophize" or "awfulize". Ellis's work with patients also became a form of cognitive therapy, known as rational emotive behaviour therapy (REBT).

Like CBT, REBT encourages patients to identify and challenge irrational negative beliefs. While REBT utilizes cognitive strategies to help clients, it also focuses on emotions and behaviours as well. In addition to identifying and disputing irrational beliefs, therapists and clients work together to target the emotional responses that accompany problematic thoughts. Clients are also encouraged to change unwanted behaviours using such tools as meditation, writing a journal, and guided imagery.

REBT can be effective in the treatment of a range of psychological disorders, including anxiety disorders and phobias, as well as specific behaviours, such as severe shyness and excessive approval-seeking.

Cosmic ordering

Essentially, cosmic ordering means asking the universe for whatever you want, and it arrives. The term was first used by Bärbel Mohr in her book *The Cosmic Ordering Service*, but the principle has been around since biblical times, when it was more often referred to as a miracle.

Although the principle of cosmic ordering is simple, it isn't easy to master without a cosmic-ordering coach to help you. A coach is able to point out how your own doubts, fears, scepticisms, jealousies, and limiting beliefs get in your way, and can give you

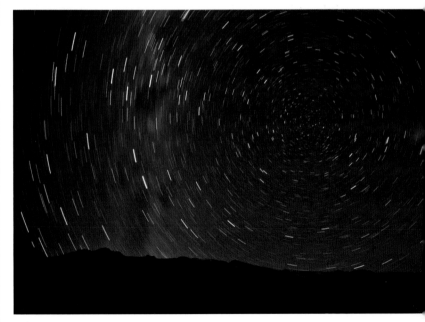

techniques to overcome these self-imposed obstacles. With the aid of a coach, you can bring more abundance into your life – whatever that means for you, and however you want that to be.

What to expect

During a one-to-one cosmic-ordering session, the coach will help you write your "wish list" and work out what you *really* want. Then you will do some work on identifying your specific limiting beliefs, which are preventing you from having the life you want; and the coach will give you techniques to de-power these.

In all probability there will be a discussion at some point during your session about making sure that your cosmic ordering does not result in others losing out. (For instance, if you ask for money, you don't want a relative to die so that you can inherit, because to gain at others' expense is bad karma.) This is often neatly covered by adding the phrase "for the good of all concerned" at the end of every cosmic order that you place, thus ensuring that no one suffers in order for you to gain.

Finally, you will look at ways to make sure that you recognize your orders when they arrive

THE LAW OF ATTRACTION

Rhonda Byrne's book *The Secret* refers to the "Law of Attraction", which is akin to cosmic ordering, while other mind–body–spirit writers, such as Wayne Dyer, refer to it as "manifesting". Whatever label you choose to give it, it's all the same thing really: it means asking the universe/Spirit/God/Allah/Source/Cosmos/Angels/Fairies/Higher Self (or whatever else you like to call it) for what you want or need, and it will come for you.

Cosmic ordering can help you to overcome limiting beliefs and fears that prevent you from having the life that you want.

(this is known as your "reticular filter"). According to the principles of cosmic ordering and the Law of Attraction (see the box on page 369), if you are generous – not necessarily just financially, but with your time, your contacts, and your attention – then you are sowing the seeds that allow the universe to work its magic. By being generous and "giving", you are effectively "paying it forward"

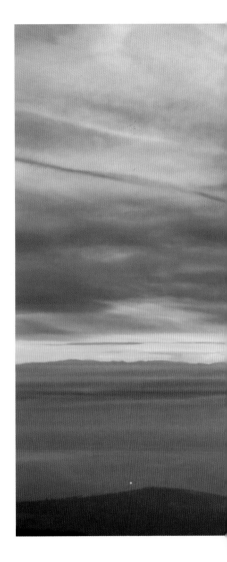

STUDY FACT

In 2006 the British television presenter and DJ Noel Edmonds credited Bärbel Mohr's book *The Cosmic Ordering Service* with turning around his career and presenting him with a new television challenge, after several years without one.

By changing the way you look at things, you can give the universe the chance to work its magic.

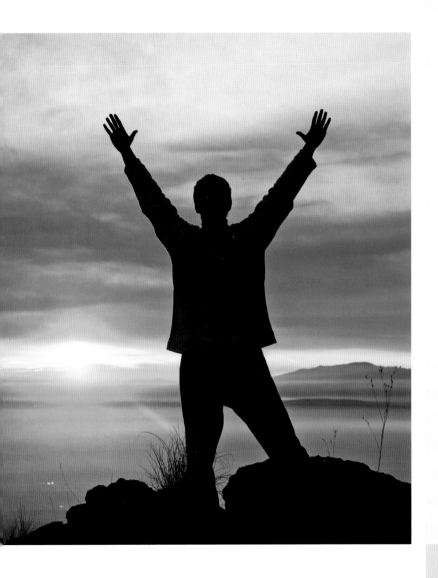

or "giving back" – whichever term you prefer – and these acts set in motion a series of acts, just like the ripples on a pond when you toss in a stone. Acts of kindness and generosity are always repaid, according to the Law of Attraction, but not always from the expected situations or quarters. Often what you give out comes back from unexpected quarters, and this is why the coach will help you to attune your reticular filter, so that you are able to discern when your cosmic ordering has delivered.

Finally, you will probably leave with an action plan, so that you can work with the universe to move you towards your goals in the coming months and years.

A session typically lasts 60–90 minutes. Some people find that one session is all they need in

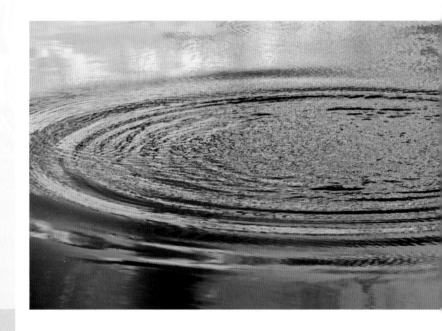

order to get "unstuck", while others prefer to return for regular coaching, or just occasionally to get an injection of motivation and direction, and to be able to work through the many and complex layers of their limiting beliefs with a professional.

Training
There is no governing body or association for cosmic ordering.

If you want to investigate further, there are several good books on the market, including *Cosmic Ordering Made Easier* by Ellen Watts, *The Secret* by Rhonda Byrne, *Wishes Fulfilled: Mastering the Art of Manifesting* by Dr Wayne Dyer, and *May Cause Miracles* by Gabrielle Bernstein. All of these authors (and others) run workshops and training sessions in cosmic ordering.

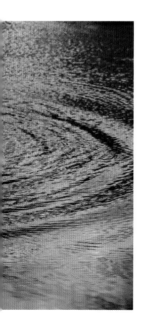

Acts of kindness and generosity can set in motion a series of effects, just like the ripples on a pond.

WRITER PROFILE

The German author **Bärbel Mohr** (1964–2010) published 20 books, including her bestselling *Bestellungen beim Universum* (*The Cosmic Ordering Service*), which has been translated into 14 languages so far, as well as a German audio edition; print sales now total more than 1.5 million copies. Initially Mohr wrote the book in 1995 for a small group of people and it was given out as a photocopy.

Quantum-field healing

Quantum-field healing (QFH) is a visualization technique in which you imagine an injury, illness, or disease as waves of energy in the quantum field, rather than as a physical thing. The process involves imagining entering the cells, going inside their DNA, shrinking in order to face atoms, going inside the atoms to meet the subatomic particles, then emerging in the quantum field, which is a field of pure energy.

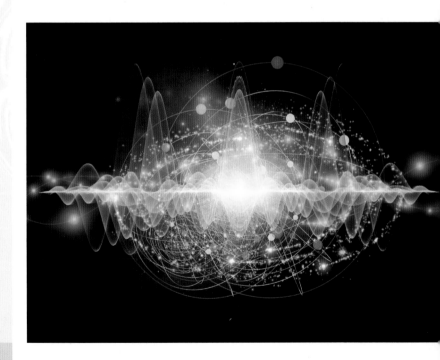

Try to imagine that, classically, healing through visualization can be brought about (at the physical level) by imagining the transformation of a physical picture of illness into a picture of wellness. With quantum-field healing you do the same, but you turn energy waves of illness into energy waves of wellness. The premise is that all physical things can be reduced to waves of energy in the quantum field.

History

Scientist and author Dr David Hamilton was researching the placebo effect, and people who recover from illness or disease through a spontaneous remission, and was relating both to the biological changes that must take place when a person with multiple-personality disorder switches personality. For instance, one personality could be allergic to orange juice and break out in hives, but the hives

Through visualization, you are able to enter the quantum field of pure energy during a quantum-field healing session.

would rapidly disappear if they switched personality to one who did not have the allergy. In all these cases, the mind is exerting considerable effects throughout the brain and body, and is doing this very quickly.

Hamilton says, "The idea for quantum-field healing came to me in the middle of the night after I had participated, first-hand, in an instant healing of a woman who'd joined a charity that some friends and I had founded. Most of the volunteers were healers of some sort. She had never heard of healing outside of the context of the Bible. After she'd been with us for a few weeks, and found out the volunteers were 'healers', she got it in her head that we were special spiritual beings sent by God to heal the world. It was the only way she could relate to it. And she thought I must be a master healer, because I was one of the initial founders of the charity."

One day, this woman was quite ill with flu. She was working on a project that could make a difference in some children's lives and was determined to finish it before going home. David continues, "I suddenly had the idea that, if she thinks I am a master healer, if I could play along, then I might be able to help facilitate a recovery. So I casually asked her if she wanted a healing. At first she was overwhelmed by the idea, because to receive a healing was a huge thing in her mind, but she eventually accepted, when I convinced her that it wouldn't drain my energy (which she was worried about). I also remarked, 'As you know, it only takes a second.' In saying this, I was trying to reinforce her belief in an instant healing that she was expecting.

"So I placed my hand on her forehead, gave her a push and blurted out, 'Cold, cancel!' She fell back and then started jumping with joy, because the flu was completely gone. It literally took about three seconds. I had simply used language and body posture to create the sense that I regularly performed such feats. It was her belief in me that resulted in her healing.

"It got me thinking more than ever before that the body really is capable of amazing things, and we just need to learn how to tap into it. Often it takes a large mental or emotional shift, certainly according to placebo, spontaneous remission, and multiple-personality disorder research.

"I realized that one way to facilitate the mental or emotional shift might be to completely change a person's perception of what an injury, illness, or disease is. Most people think of these things as physical and relatively long-lasting, but if you shift your perspective and consider them from a quantum perspective, they are really just waves of energy, and waves of energy can change rapidly. I hoped that a shift like this might break through a person's normal perception of illness or disease and thus tap into the ability the body has of changing quickly."

Who can benefit?

People use QFH for all manner of different situations, from physical conditions to emotional issues, where they imagine changing the energy waves of an emotion or belief. It is especially good for people who are experiencing pain, with sufferers often reporting an easing or disappearance of pain at workshops.

What to expect

QFH comprises a simple 15–20-minute visualization that you can do by yourself or for someone else, by placing your hands upon them. You can even do the technique at a distance.

Training

Currently the only practitioner is Dr David Hamilton. However, he has taught many people the technique, and they use it as and when they wish. You can learn QFH from his CD, his book *How Your Mind Can Heal Your Body* (which contains the relevant script), or at one of his workshops.

David also teaches an advanced version, called Time-Displaced Quantum Field Healing, in which you basically imagine shifting back through time at the quantum level to the point in space and time where the possibility of the present illness, disease, or condition first arose. During the course you initially learn some science about the nature of time, including quantum-physics research, which demonstrates that choices in the present really do influence conditions in the past.

STUDY FACT

The inspiration that led Dr Hamilton (who has a first-class honours degree in chemistry and a PhD in organic chemistry) to form his unique fusion of science and spirituality came from his time working for the pharmaceutical giant AstraZeneca. When testing new medicines he was amazed that although you might get 75 per cent of people improving on a particular drug, it's not uncommon to get 50–74 per cent improving on a placebo. For him, this was compelling evidence of the power of the mind.

Biodynamic therapy

Developed more than 50 years ago by the Norwegian clinical psychologist, psychotherapist, and physiotherapist Gerda Boyesen (1922–2005), biodynamic therapy uses a variety of different techniques to restore someone to their natural, exuberant, spontaneous self.

The term "biodynamic" refers to the free-flowing life energy that moves naturally around a healthy body – something we should all experience. But, over time, this flow of energy becomes disturbed, depending on how we deal with life events. The more distorted it is, the less healthy we feel, physically or psychologically. Our life story gets shown in our body, by our posture, muscle tone, and face shape. As life knocks us, we inhibit our natural self-expression, often keeping unexpressed feelings inside us, where it gets stored in muscle groups, creating blockage and pain.

By adding bodywork, in the form of deep, gentle, or powerful massage (as needed), to more traditional psychotherapy and psychology, this holistic healing method not only breaks down the barriers and blocks in the mind, but also works to release stress and tension stored in the body. This reconnects us to what is known in biodynamic psychology as the Primary Personality – your vibrant core self, unaffected by life's challenges – which in turn clears the way towards living an authentic, fulfilling life.

Who can benefit?

This enlightening and deep healing process benefits anyone who wants to be free of stress-related symptoms, such as headaches, anxiety, and insomnia, as well as depression, ME, and arthritis. Biodynamic therapy can boost the metabolism, bring peace and calm to shattered nerves, balance the respiratory system, and ease tension and pain in the back, neck, and shoulder muscles.

It helps those in pain or under pressure for whatever reason, as well as those who want their lives to flow and feel joyful again. If you're on a path of self-discovery and want help uncovering and healing the things that are holding you back, then biodynamic therapy can dramatically help.

This therapy is increasingly being applied in the fields of trauma recovery, conflict resolution, pre- and post-operative care, and, more recently, with women who are recovering from the effects of domestic and other forms of violence. Biodynamic methods are currently being established in a new branch of medicine known as "biodynamic medicine" and are being applied in the treatment of potentially all diagnosed conditions, at all stages of a person's life.

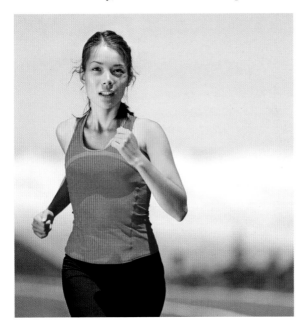

Biodynamic therapy can help you to feel more joyful and energetic again.

What to expect

After an initial consultation at which you will discuss your reasons for treatment, your symptoms, lifestyle, and diet, subsequent sessions are different, depending on what you need, and what you and your practitioner mutually decide is right at that moment. Traditional psychotherapy is always a part of the process, so expect to talk about your emotions and issues, as well as having your non-verbal language observed – for instance, your eye expression, the sound of your voice, and other gestures that reveal communication between the conscious and subconscious.

In one session you may spend the whole time talking, while in another session you may be lying down, fully clothed, breathing deeply as you let your emotions rise, which may make you feel like punching your fists into the mattress underneath you or crying your eyes out. It is all done with

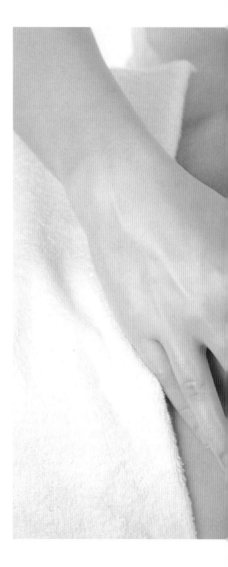

Specifically tailored massage can be used in addition to traditional psychotherapy and breathing techniques.

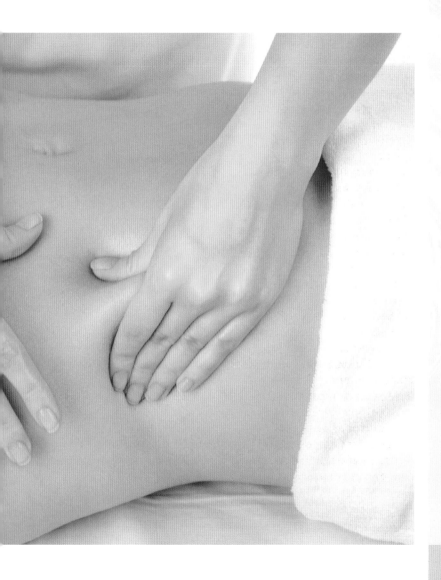

gentle compassion, care, and at the client's pace.

Biodynamic massage also plays a big part in the treatment, whereby your therapist gives you a tailored massage on bare skin or fully clothed (your choice), because either is effective at helping the body release deeply held emotions and tension. During the massage, a loudspeaker stethoscope monitors the sounds of the small intestine, so that the practitioner can support the body's own method of eliminating emotional stress by engaging "psycho-peristalsis" through specialized touch. Boyesen concluded that massage could release unwanted feelings and emotions, and that this release would involve similar sounds coming from the intestines to those made during digestion; and she named these noises psycho-peristalsis.

Usually you will have a course of weekly or fortnightly meetings, after which you may experience a complete spiritual transformation, find the courage to aim for new challenges in your career or lifestyle, and become who you really are, underneath all the layers covering up your true self.

According to Mary Molloy, founder and principal of the Institute of Biodynamic Medicine (formerly the Gerda Boyesen International Institute of Biodynamic Psychology and Psychotherapy), "Clients can develop a new and keen interest in nutrition, different communication skills, end dysfunctional relationships, establish or revive fulfilling relationships . . . they begin to experience synchronicity and esoteric aspects of life, and many develop an interest in natural remedies and the whole world of soul and spirit."

Training

Through the website of the Institute of Biodynamic Medicine (see page 391) you can find details of the various options that are available, including ongoing one-to-one sessions at biodynamic clinics in the UK and Ireland; individually tailored residential programmes, of 5–30

ELIMINATING EMOTIONAL STRESS

As Gerda Boyesen discovered, after years of research and practice, the process of storing emotion in the body particularly affects the muscles in the gut, which are majorly involved in our self-regulation of conflict and stress. In biodynamic therapy, special attention is paid to the sounds the stomach makes, because, in addition to being related to digestion, these are also connected to an independent internal motion (now known as a "migrating motor complex") that responds to touch and acts as a clear signal as to whether or not you are releasing emotional blocks.

Boyesen's findings followed on from the work of Wilhelm Reich (a student of Sigmund Freud), showing the importance of the body and the power of touch in psychotherapy, and are confirmed by new research into cell biology and neuroscience. Aspects of the biodynamic approach include Eastern philosophy and medicine, bioenergetics, energy medicine, and current findings in medicine and science.

days, in Killala, County Mayo, Ireland; group, introductory, and specialized retreats; plus a ten-day Annual International Biodynamic Summer School.

The institute also trains people to postgraduate level in this field, and gets biodynamic psychotherapists and practitioners fully qualified, via a four-year, part-time diploma course in the field of biodynamic psychology and the related treatments developed by Boyesen. If you are a nurse, social worker, teacher, psychologist, psychotherapist, holistic practitioner, healthcare worker, or other professional, you can undertake a foundation course in biodynamic skills, to incorporate this therapy into your current healing career.

Useful contacts

GENERAL

Complementary and Natural Healthcare Council (CNHC) – www.cnhc.org.uk

European Federation for Complementary and Alternative Medicine – www.efcam.eu

Institute of Complementary and Natural Medicine (ICNM) – www.icnm.org.uk

National Center for Complementary and Integrative Health – www.nccih.nih.gov

1 CLASSIC THERAPIES

American Acupuncture Council – www.acupuncturecouncil.com

American Association of Acupuncture and Oriental Medicine – www.aaaomonline.org

British Acupuncture Council – www.acupuncture.org.uk

Council for Soft Tissue Therapies – www.gcmt.org.uk

National Association of Massage and Manipulative Therapists – www.nammt.co.uk

Aromatherapy Council – www.facebook.com/pages/Aromatherapy-Council/141638522588552?sk=info&tab=page_info

International Federation of Aromatherapists – www.ifaroma.org

National Association for Holistic Aromatherapy – www.naha.org

American Institute of Homeopathy – www.homeopathyusa.org

British Homeopathic Association – www.britishhomeopathic.org

European Central Council of Homeopaths – www.homeopathy-ecch.org

European Committee for Homeopathy (medical doctors with homeopathy qualifications) – www.homeopathyeurope.org

National Center for Homeopathy – www.nationalcenterforhomeopathy.org

North American Society of Homeopaths – www.homeopathy.org

Society of Homeopaths – www.homeopathy-soh.org

American Osteopathic Association – www.osteopathic.org

European Federation of Osteopaths – www.efo.eu

General Osteopathic Council – www.osteopathy.org.uk

International Academy of Osteopathy – www.osteopathie.eu

American Chiropractic Association – www.acatoday.org

European Academy of Chiropractic – www.eacacademy.com

General Chiropractic Council – www.gcc-uk.org

International Chiropractors Association – www.chiropractic.org

American Association of Professional Hypnotherapists – www.aaph.org

American Hypnosis Association –
www.hypnosis.edu/aha

European Society of Hypnosis –
www.esh-hypnosis.eu

General Hypnotherapy Register –
www.general-hypnotherapy-register.com

General Hypnotherapy Standards
Council – www.general-hypnotherapy-register.com

National Hypnotherapy Society –
www.nationalhypnotherapysociety.org

American Herbalists' Guild –
www.americanherbalistsguild.com

European Herbal and Traditional
Medicine Practitioners Association –
www.ehtpa.eu

Medicines and Healthcare Products
Regulatory Agency – www.mhra.gov.uk

National Institute of Medical
Herbalists – www.nimh.org.uk

North American Institute of Medical
Herbalism – www.naimh.com

International Association of Reiki
Professionals – www.iarpreiki.org

International Center for Reiki Training
– www.reiki.org

Reiki Alliance – www.reikialliance.com

Reiki Association –
www.reikiassociation.net

Reiki Council – www.reikicouncil.org.uk

UK Reiki Federation – www.reikifed.co.uk

Association of Reflexologists –
www.aor.org.uk

British Association for Applied
Nutrition and Nutritional Therapy –
www.bant.org.uk

Nutritional Therapy Association –
www.nutritionaltherapy.com

Nutritional Therapy Council –
www.nutritionaltherapycouncil.org.uk

Nutritional Therapy
Education Commission –
www.nteducationcommission.org.uk

Wholistic Nutritional Medicine Society –
www.wnms.org.uk

2 MULTIDISCIPLINARY HEALING SYSTEMS

American Academy of
Ayurvedic Medicine –
www.ayurvedicacademy.com

Ayurvedic Practitioners Association –
www.apa.uk.com

British Association of Accredited
Ayurvedic Practitioners –
www.britayurpractitioners.com/
about-baaap.html

European Ayurveda Medical Association –
www.ayurveda-association.eu

National Ayurvedic Medical
Association – www.ayurvedanama.org

American TCM Society –
www.atcms.org

Association of Traditional Chinese
Medicine and Acupuncture UK –
www.atcm.co.uk

European Traditional Chinese
Medicine Association –
www.etcma.org

American Association of Naturopathic
Physicians – www.naturopathic.org

American Naturopathic Medical
Association – www.anma.org

American Naturopaths' Association –
www.americannaturopaths
association.com

Association for Natural Medicine in Europe – www.anme-ngo.eu

Association of Naturopathic Practitioners – www.naturopathy-anp.com

Association of Registered Colon Hydrotherapists – www.colonic-association.org

British Naturopathic Association – www.naturopaths.org.uk

British Naturopathic and Osteopathic Association – www.bnoa.org.uk

College of Naturopathic Medicine – www.naturopathy-uk.com

General Council and Register of Naturopaths – www.gcrn.org.uk

General Naturopathic Council – www.gncouncil.co.uk

American Polarity Therapy Association – www.polaritytherapy.org

International Polarity Education Alliance – www.polarityeducation.org

UK Polarity Therapy Association – www.polarity.tk

3 POSTURAL/BODYWORK TECHNIQUES

American Society for the Alexander Technique – www.amsatonline.org

Professional Association of Alexander Teachers (PAATT) – www.paat.org.uk

Society of Teachers of the Alexander Technique (STAT) – www.stat.org.uk

European and Israeli Feldenkrais Training and Accreditation Board (EuroTAB) – www.eurotab.org

Feldenkrais Guild UK – www.feldenkrais.co.uk

Feldenkrais Guild of North America – www.feldenkrais.com

Feldenkrais International Training Centre – www.feldenkrais-itc.com

American Dance Therapy Association – www.adta.org

Association of Dance Movement – www.admt.org.uk

European Association Dance Movement Therapy – www.eadmt.com

European Rolfing Association – www.rolfing.org

Rolf Institute of Structural Integration – www.rolf.org

American Bowen Academy – www.americanbowen.academy

Bowen Therapy Professional Association (BTPA) – www.bowentherapy.org.uk

American CranioSacral Therapy Association – www.upledger.com

Biodynamic Cranialsacral Therapy Association of North America – www.craniosacraltherapy.org

Craniosacral Therapy Association – www.craniosacral.co.uk

International Cranial Association – www.icra-uk.org

International Shiatsu Network – www.shiatsunetwork.com

Shiatsu Society – www.shiatsusociety.org

American Organization for Bodywork Therapies of Asia – www.aobta.org

British Health Qigong Association – www.healthqigong.org.uk

Health Qigong Federation UK – www.healthqigong.co.uk

National (USA) Qigong Association – www.nqa.org

Infinite Tai Chi – www.infinitetaichi.com

Tai Chi Union for Great Britain – www.taichiunion.com

Taijiquan and Qi Gong Federation for Europe – www.tcfe.org

Taoist Tai Chi Association of the USA – www.taoist.org/usa/

Tui Na UK – www.tuinauk.com

UK Register of Tui na Chinese Massage – www.ukrtcm.org

World Tui-na Association – www.tui-na.com

4 BREATHING TECHNIQUES

British Rebirth Society – www.rebirthingbreathwork.co.uk

Rebirther Training: Avalon Institute of Rebirthing (AIR) – www.rebirther.co.uk

Rebirther Training: Lovesbreath Trainings – www.lovesbreath.co.uk

Rebirthing Breathwork International – www.rebirthingbreathwork.com

Transformational Breath Foundation UK – www.transformationalbreath.co.uk

Buteyko Breathing Association – www.buteykobreathing.org

International Association of Buteyko Practitioners – www.iaobp.org

Global Professional Breathwork Alliance (GPBA) – www.breathworkalliance.com

Stanislav and Christina Grof Foundation (formerly the Association for Holotropic Breathwork International) – www.groffoundation.org

Holotropic Breathwork – www.grof-holotropic-breathwork.net

International Breathwork Foundation (IBF) – www.ibfnetwork.com

Holographic Breathing (Martin Jones) – www.holographic-breathing.com

5 HEALING THROUGH THE SENSES

American Art Therapy Association – www.arttherapy.org

International Art Therapy Organization – www.internationalarttherapy.org

British Association of Art Therapists – www.baat.org

European Consortium for Art Therapies Education – www.ecarte.info

Aura-Soma – www.aura-soma.com

Guild of Naturopathic Iridologists International – www.gni-international.org

International Iridology Practitioners Association – www.iridologyassn.org

Bates Method International – www.seeing.org

Visions of Joy – www.visionsofjoy.org

British Academy of Sound Therapy – www.healthysound.com

College of Sound Healing – www.collegeofsoundhealing.co.uk

International Association of Sound Therapy – www.soundtherapyassociation.org

Pineal Toning – www.pineal-tones.com/pinealtones

Sound Healers Association – www.soundhealersassociation.org

Sound Therapy Association – www.soundtherapyassn.org.uk

Aquatic Therapy Association of Chartered Physiotherapists – www.csp.org.uk/professional-networks/atacp

Dr Emoto (hydrotherapy; for free download of children's book) – www.masaru-emoto.net and www.emoto-peace-project.com

North American Association for Light Therapy – www.naalt.org

Seasonal Affective Disorder Association – www.sada.org.uk

British Association of Flower Essence Producers (BAFEP) – www.bafep.com

British Flower and Vibrational Essences Association (BFVEA) – www.bfvea.com

Flower Essence Society – www.flowersociety.org

Flowersense (Clare G. Harvey) – www.flowersense.co.uk

La Vie de la Rose Flower Essences – www.laviedelarose.com

British Association for Music Therapy – www.bamt.org

Music Therapy Charity – www.musictherapy.org.uk

Biomagnetic Therapy Association – www.biomagnetic.org

Magnetic Therapy Council – www.magnetictherapyfacts.org

National Acupuncture Detoxification Association (NADA) (auricular acupuncture) – www.acudetox.com

Society of Auricular Acupuncturists – www.auricularacupuncture.org.uk

6 ENERGY OR VIBRATIONAL HEALING

Affiliation of Crystal Healing Organisations – www.crystal-healing.org

American Society of Dowsers – www.dowsers.org

British Society of Dowsers – www.britishdowsers.org

Crystal Therapy Council – www.crystalcouncil.org

Institute of Crystal and Gem Therapists – www.icgt.co.uk

American Kinesiology Association – www.americankinesiology.org

Association of Systematic Kinesiology – www.systematic-kinesiology.co.uk

Kinesiology Federation – www.kinesiologyfederation.co.uk

Angelic Reiki Association – www.angelicreikiassociation.co.uk

Angelic Reiki Foundation – www.angelic-reiki.org

International Angelic Reiki
Foundation –
www.angelicreikimagic.com

Energy Medicine (Donna Eden) –
www.innersource.net

Reconnective Healing –
www.thereconnection.com

BodyTalk System™ –
www.bodytalksystem.com

Zimbaté Healing –
www.zimbatehealing.com

Divine Empowerment –
www.divineempowerment.co.uk

Metatronic Healing® –
www.metatronic-life.com

Quantum-Touch® –
www.quantumtouch.com

Quantum Touch (UK practitioners) –
www.thehealingtouch.uk.com

The Journey (Brandon Bays) –
www.thejourney.com

ThetaHealing® – www.thetahealing.com

7 PROGRESSION AND REGRESSION THERAPIES

Past and Future Life Society –
www.pflsociety.org

Past Life Regression Academy –
www.regressionacademy.com

Past Life Therapists Association –
www.pastliferegression.co.uk

Past Reality Integration International –
www.pastrealityintegration.com

Lorraine Flaherty
(future-life progression) –
www.innerjourneys.co.uk

Anne Jirsch (future-life progression) –
www.annejirsch.com

Center for Akashic Studies (Linda
Howe) – www.akashicstudies.com

Amanda Romania (Akashic Records) –
www.amandaromania.com

Soul Realignment (Akashic Records) –
www.soulrealignment.com

8 MIND AND PSYCHOLOGICAL TECHNIQUES

International Sophrology Federation –
www.sophrologyinternational.org

American Meditation Society –
www.americanmeditationsociety.org

British Meditation Society –
www.britishmeditationsociety.org

International Meditation
Teachers Association –
www.meditationteachers.org

Meditation Society of America –
www.meditationsociety.com

Mindfulness Meditation –
www.bemindful.co.uk

American Group Psychotherapy
Association – www.agpa.org

American Psychological Association –
www.apa.org

American Psychotherapy Association –
www.americanpsychotherapy.com

Association for the Advancement of
Gestalt Therapy – www.aagt.org

British Association for Counselling
and Psychotherapy – www.bacp.co.uk

British Psychological Society – www.bps.org.uk

European Association for Body Psychotherapy – www.eabp.org

European Association for Counselling – www.eac.eu.com

European Association for Psychotherapy – www.europsyche.org

European Association for Gestalt Therapy – www.eagt.org

Gestalt Psychotherapy and Training Institute – www.gpti.org.uk

UK Council for Psychotherapy (UKCP) – www.psychotherapy.org.uk and www.ukcp.org.uk

United States Association for Body Psychotherapy – www.usabp.org

American Board of NLP – www.abh-abnlp.com

Association for NLP – www.anlp.org

Energetic NLP – www.energeticnlp.com

International Association for Neuro-Linguistic Programming – www.ia-nlp.org

International NLP Trainers Association – www.inlpta.co.uk

Association for the Advancement of Meridian Energy Techniques (AAMET) – www.aamet.org

EFT Centre (co-founders: Sue Beer and Emma Roberts) – www.theeftcentre.com

Picture-tapping Technique – www.healingspiritwithin.co.uk

Matrix Reimprinting practitioners – www.matrixreimprinting.com

Compassionate Mind Foundation – www.compassionatemind.co.uk

F**k It Therapy – www.thefuckitlife.com

American Institute for Cognitive Therapy – www.cognitivetherapynyc.com

Beating the Blues (CBT) – www.beatingtheblues.co.uk

Beck Institute for Cognitive Behavior Therapy – beckinstitute.org

European Association for Behavioural and Cognitive Therapies – www.eabct.eu

FearFighter (CBT) – www.fearfighter.com

Association for Behavioral and Cognitive Therapies – www.abct.org

Living Life to the Full (CBT) – www.livinglifetothefull.com

National Association of Cognitive-Behavioral Therapists – www.nacbt.org

Association of Cosmic Ordering Practitioners – www.cosmicordering.net

Quantum-field Healing – www.drdavidhamilton.com

Institute of Biodynamic Medicine – www.biodynamic.org

Index

5Rhythms® 105, 107

A
Academy of Systematic
    Kinesiology 232
acupuncture 11, 18–19,
    80, 135
    acupressure for children
    19, 21
    auricular acupuncture
    226
    history 19
    moxibustion 22–3
    what to expect 19–20
    who can benefit? 19
Akashic Record therapy
    310–11
    history 311–12
    training 315
    what to expect 314–15
    who can benefit? 312–14
Alexander Technique
    96, 109
    healer profile 97
    training 99
    what to expect 96–9
    who can benefit? 96
Alexander, Frederick
    Matthias 97, 167
American Dance Therapy
    Association 107
American Herbalists
    Guild 57
American Polarity Therapy
    Association 92, 93
anatripsis 24
angelic reiki 238
    guided by angels 241
    history 238–41

self-help 243
    training 242–3
    what to expect 241–2
Angelic Reiki Association
    242
aromatherapy 11, 26, 30–1
    caution 32
    essential oils 30, 31, 33
    history 31–2
    training 33
    who can benefit? 32–3
art therapy 170
    caution 172
    history 171
    what to expect 171–2
    who can benefit? 171
Association for Neuro-
    Linguistic Programming
    (ANLP) 337–8
Aura-Soma® 178–9
auricular therapy 225
    auricular acupuncture
    226
    thermo-auricular therapy
    228–9
    training 227
    what to expect 227
    who can benefit? 227
Australian Acupuncture
    and Chinese Medicine
    Association 84
Ayurveda 12, 74–5
    Ayurvedic medicine
    76, 180
    history 75
    marma massage 28–9,
    77–8
    training 79
    Vedic astrology 78

what to expect 76–9
    who can benefit? 75–6

B
Ba Duan Jin 128
Bach, Edward 211, 213, 215
Bailey, Alice 311–12
Bandler, Richard 335
Bates method 185
    eye basics 187
    history 185–7
    pinhole glasses 188
    relaxation 190
Bates, W. H. *Perfect Sight
    Without Glasses* 185
Bays, Brandon 10, 284, 285, 286
Beardall, Alan 235
Beck, Aaron 364, 367
Bernstein, Gabrielle 373
Bible 32
biodynamic therapy 378
    eliminating emotional
    stress 383
    training 382–3
    what to expect 380–2
    who can benefit? 378–9
Blair, Ellie 264
Blake-Wilson, Pamela 177
Blavatsky, Helena 279, 311
BodyTalk System™ 10, 250
    healer profile 252–3
    self-help 251
    what to expect 251
    who can benefit? 250–1
Borland, Denise 149, 150
Bosch, Ingeborg 301–2
Bowen therapy 113
    asking the body to
    change 113

Bowen for children and
  pets 115
case-study 114
history 113
what to expect 114–15
who can benefit 113–14
Bowen, Tom 113, 115
Boyesen, Gerda 378, 382, 383
British Academy of Sound
  Therapy (BAST) 192,
  193, 194
British Association of Art
  Therapists (BAAT) 171, 172
Brown, Elizabeth 257
Brown, Michael 149
Buteyko 151
  Buteyko for children 155
  caution 151
  history 152
  self-help 154
  training 155
  what to expect 154–5
  who can benefit? 152–4
Buteyko, Konstantin 152
Butler, Brian 232
Byrne, Rhonda *The Secret*
  369, 373

C
Cayce, Edgar 312
Caycedo, Alfonson 318
Center for Disease Control
  and Prevention 285
Chace, Marian 105–7
chakra healing 276
  crown chakra 281
  heart chakra 280–1
  history 276–9
  root chakra 279
  sacral chakra 279–80
  solar-plexus chakra 280
  third-eye or brow chakra
  281

throat chakra 281
what to expect 282–3
who can benefit? 279
chakras 10, 176–8
Chan, Jason 132
chi kung *see* qigong
children
  acupressure for children 21
  Bowen Therapy 115
  Buteyko 155
  chiropractic 44–5
  cranio-sacral therapy 118
  picture-tapping
    technique (PTT) for
    children 348
  tui na Chinese massage
  138
chiropractic 43
  history 44
  training 46
  what to expect 45–7
  who can benefit? 44–5
Chopra, Deepak 149, 285
cognitive behaviour therapy
  (CBT) 328, 334, 363
  healer profile 364
  self-help 365
  training 365–7
  what to expect 363–5
  who can benefit? 363
colonic hydrotherapy 88
colour therapy 173–4
  chakras 176–8
  dyslexia 174
  self-help 177
  what to expect 175–6
  who can benefit 174
compassion-focused
  therapy (CFT) 353–4
  compassionate mind
    training (CMT) 357
  emotion-regulation
    systems 355

healer profile 353
training 357
what to expect 356
who can benefit? 356
Compassionate Mind
  Foundation 357
Cooper, Lyz 192
Core, Christine and Kevin
  238–40, 241
  Angelic Reiki 243
cosmic ordering 368–9
  Law of Attraction 369
  training 373
  what to expect 369–73
  writer profile 373
Coué, Emile 325
counselling 93, 119
Craig, Gary 339, 343
craniosacral therapy (CST)
  116–17
  training 119
  what to expect 119
  who can benefit 117–19
  working with the whole
    person 117
crystals 10
cupping 136, 137, 138

D
dance movement therapy 105
  caution 108
  history 105–7
  what to expect 108
  who can benefit? 108
Daoism 131, 133–4
Davis, Philip 344
Dawson, Karl 349
Dean, Liz 241, 242
Dennison, Paul 235
Dewe, Bruce 235
divine empowerment 262
  energetic "apps" 263
  what to expect 263–4

dowsing therapy 254
    distance dowsing 256
    healer profile 257
    training 255
    what to expect 254–5
Dyer, Wayne 369, 373
dyslexia 174

E

Eden, Donna 244, 245,
    248, 249
Edmonds, Noel 370
electromagnetic-field
    therapy 220, 222–3
Elizabeth II 34
Ellis, Albert 367
emotional freedom
    techniques (EFT) 339,
    344, 346, 349, 352
    history 339
    training 343
    using a practitioner
    342–3
    what to expect 341–2
    who can benefit? 339–41
Emoto, Masaru 200–1, 202
Energetic NLP™ 338
energy medicine 244
    healer profile 245
    self-help 248
    training 249
    two levels of help 247
    what to expect 248–9
Erickson, Milton 335
Esdaile, James 48–9
essential oils 30
    popular essential oils and
    their uses 33
    what are essential oils?
    31
eurythmy 105
External Qi Healing (EQH)
    128

F

F**k It therapy 358–9
    F**k It retreat 360–1
    Gaia's magic 362
    healer profile 358
    what to expect 359
    who can benefit? 359
Feldenkrais Method® 100–1
    Feldenkrais® Practitioner
    Training 104
    healer profile 100
    training 104
    what to expect 101–4
    who can benefit? 101
Feldenkrais, Moshe 100,
    101, 167
Fitzgerald, William 65
Flaherty, Lorraine 304–6
Food and Drug
    Administration (FDA) 57
Freud, Sigmund 171, 331, 383
future-life progression 304
    self-help 306
    training 309
    what to expect 306–9
    who can benefit? 304–6

G

Gabriel, Clare 144, 145, 146
General Chiropractic
    Council 46
Gestalt therapy 332–3
Gilbert, Paul 353, 356
Giser, Art 338
Global Inspiration
    Conference (GIC) 146
Global Professional
    Breathwork Alliance
    (GPBA) 146
Goldberg, Bruce 304
Goodheart, George 232,
    234–5, 237
Gordon, Richard 271, 273

Grinder, John 335
Grof Transpersonal
    Training 163
Grof, Stanislav and Christina
    156, 159, 162
gua sha 137, 138

H

Hahnemann, Samuel 34
Hamilton, David 375–6, 377
Hammer, Michael 241
Harman, Antonia 262, 263
Harvey, Clare 211
Hawn, Goldie 149
healing therapies 8–10
    costs 15
    finding a therapist 13–15
    innovative techniques
    10–12
    medical advice 15
    using this book 13
Heller, Joseph 112
Hellerwork 112
Herbal and Traditional
    Medicine Practitioners
    Association 57
herbal liniments 137
herbal medicine 11, 53, 135
    caution 55
    Chinese herbal medicine
    80, 84
    industry regulation 56
    private insurance 57
    training 56–7
    what to expect 54–6
    who can benefit? 54
Hippocrates 85
holographic breathing 164
    how to breathe
    holographically 166
    training 167
    what to expect 167
    who can benefit? 164–7

Holotropic Breathwork™ 156–8
  caution 159
  healer profile 162
  how often? 161
  training 163
  what to expect 160–3
  who can benefit? 158–9
homeopathy 11, 34–5
  home first-aid kits 37
  homeopathic designations 35
  training 37
  what to expect 36–7
  who can benefit? 35–6
Hopi ear-candle therapy 228–9
Horowitz, Leonard 193
Howe, Linda 315
hydrotherapy 197
  colonic hydrotherapy 88
  healer profile 200–1
  healing minerals 199
  what to expect 198–9
  who can benefit? 198
hypnotherapy 47–8
  caution 50
  history 48–9
  hypnotherapy and labour 52
  training 52
  what to expect 50–2
  who can benefit? 49–50

I
IFVM Flower School 211
Infinite Chi Kung™ 132
Infinite Tai Chi™ 132
Ingham, Eunice 65–6
Innersource 248, 249
Institute of Biodynamic Medicine 382

International Breathwork Foundation (IBF) 146
International College of Kinesiology 234
International Polarity Education Alliance 93
International Water for Life Foundation 201
Intuitive Colorimeter 174
iridology 86–7, 180–1
  dominant eye 183
  what to expect 181–4

J
Jackson-Main, Peter Practical Iridology 183
jaundice, infantile 209
Jin Shin Jyutsu 124
Jirsch, Anne The Future is Yours 306
Jones, Martin 164, 167
Jung, Carl 105, 171

K
Kerr, Catherine 327
kinesiology 232
  applied and systematic kinesiology 232
  classical kinesiology and diversification 237
  healer profile 234–5
  history 232
  training 236
  what to expect 235–6
  who can benefit? 234–5
Kinesiology Federation 235
Korte, Andreas 210
Kravitz, Judith 150

L
Laban, Rudolf 105
Laozi 125
Law of Attraction 351, 369, 372

Leadbeater, Charles Webster 279, 311
Light Foundation 132
light therapy 203
  caution 203, 207
  precautions 206
  PUVA therapy 203–4
  seasonal affective disorder 208
  UVB therapy 203–4
  what to expect 204–9
  who can benefit? 204
Ling Chi Healing Art™ 132
Ling, Per Henrik 24
Lipton, Bruce 285

M
magnet therapy 220
  magnet efficacy and strengths 223–4
  what to expect 223
  who can benefit? 220–3
Maharishi Mahesh 324
Manual Lymphatic Drainage 120–2
marma massage 28–9, 77–8
massage therapy 24
  history 24
  marma massage 28–9, 77–8
  massage with a partner 26
  self-massage 27
  what to expect 25–6
  who can benefit? 25
matrix reimprinting (MR) 349–51
  what to expect 352
  who can benefit? 351–2
Mawang-diu Silk Texts 125
McKann, Katie 167
Medical Research Council (MRC) 174

Medicines and Healthcare Products Regulatory Agency (MHRA) 56–7
meditation 143, 322
  auto-suggestion 325
  mindfulness meditation 11, 326–7
  training 325
  Transcendental Meditation (TM) 322, 324
  vipassana meditation 325
  what to expect 322–4
  Zen meditation 324
Mental Health Foundation 326
Merivale, Philippa 266, 267, 268
Metatronic Healing® 266
  Metatron's role 268–9
  training 270
  what to expect 267–70
  who can benefit? 266–7
Miller, Hamish 256
mindfulness meditation 11, 326–7
mineral waters 199
Mohr, Bärbel *The Cosmic Ordering Service* 368, 370, 373
Molloy, Mary 382
moxibustion 22, 137
  caution 23
  self-help 22–3
music therapy 216
  research 218
  training 219
  what to expect 218–19
  who can benefit? 216–18

N
National Institute for Health and Care Excellence (NICE) 328

National Institute of Medical Herbalists 57
naturopathy 85–6
  causes of illness 89
  colonic hydrotherapy 88
  infections 86
  training 88
  what to expect 86–8
  who can benefit? 86
neuro-linguistic programming (NLP) 335–7, 343
  Energetic NLP™ 338
  training 337–8
  what to expect 337
  who can benefit? 337
neuro-linguistic psychotherapy 335
new-generation flower essences 10, 210–12
  healer profiles 211, 213, 215
  self-help 212
  what to expect 214–15
  who can benefit? 212–14
nutritional therapy 69
  caution 70
  training 70
  what to expect 70
  who can benefit? 69–70

O
Orr, leonard 144
osteopathy 38
  caution 40
  history 39
  referrals 42
  training 42
  what to expect 40–2
  who can benefit? 39–40

P
Palmer, Daniel David 44
palming 190

paradigm shift of 2012 9–10, 276, 279
Parkin, John C and Gaia 358, 360–1, 362
Past and Future Life Society 309
past-life integration therapy 300–1
  history 301–2
  self-help 302
  what to expect 302–3
  who can benefit? 302
past-life readings 298
past-life regression therapy 11, 296
  caution 296
  genetic memory 298
  imagination 298
  reincarnation 298
  relationships 299
  soul memory 298
  what are past-life experiences? 298
  what to expect 299
  who can benefit? 298–9
Peace Project 201, 202
Perls, Fritz 332, 335
Pert, Candace B. 285
pets
  Bowen therapy 115
picture-tapping technique (PTT) 344–5
  PTT for children 348
  what to expect 346–8
  who can benefit? 346
Pilates 283
pineal toning 196
pinhole glasses 188
polarity therapy 90
  awareness/counselling 93
  bodywork 91–3
  diets and nutritional advice 93

healer profile 92
polarity yoga 93
what to expect 91–3
who can benefit? 90–1
Presence Process 149
psychotherapy 119, 143, 158, 328
  Gestalt therapy 332–3
  psychodynamic psychotherapy 119, 331
  psychosis 328
  training 334
  what to expect 331–4
  who can benefit? 328–31
pulsed electromagnetic-field therapy (PEMFT) 222–3

Q
qigong 80, 83, 125–6, 135
  nei gong/tao yin 125
  what to expect 127–8
  who can benefit? 126–7
quantum-field healing (QFH) 374–5
  history 375–6
  Time-Displaced Quantum Field Healing 377
  training 377
  what to expect 377
  who can benefit? 376–7
Quantum-Touch 271–2
  healer profile 273
  training 272–5
  what to expect 272
  who can benefit? 272

R
rational emotive behaviour therapy (RABT) 367
rebirthing breathwork 143–4
  history 144
  training 146

what to expect 145–6
  who can benefit? 144–5
reflexology 64
  healer profile 65
  history 65–6
  training 68
  what to expect 67–8
  who can benefit? 66–7
Register of Tui Na Chinese Massage 138
Reich, Wilhelm 105, 383
reiki 58–9, 258–60, 271
  higher levels 62
  history 59
  training 62–3
  what to expect 60–2
  who can benefit? 59–60
Rolf, Ida 109
Rolfing 24, 109–10, 112
  temporary painfulness 110
  what to expect 110–11
  who can benefit? 110
Romania, Amanda *Akashic Therapy* 311
Roth, Gabrielle 105, 107

S
Satir, Virginia 335
Schotte, Natalia 215
sclerology 184
Scott, Jimmy 235
seasonal affective disorder (SAD) 208
Seichem 63
shiatsu 24, 120
  pressure points 122
  training 124
  what to expect 122–3
  who can benefit? 120–2
Shiatsu Society 124
Sinnett, Alfred Percy *Esoteric Buddhism* 311

Snyder, Carolyn 258, 259, 261
Society of Teachers of the Alexander Technique 99
Solfeggio tuning 193
sophrology 318–19
  self-help 321
  what to expect 320–1
  who can benefit? 319–20
Soul Wisdom healing 300
sound frequencies 195
Stanislav and Christina Grof Foundation 163
Steiner, Rudolf 312
Stibal, Vianna 10, 288, 291
Still, Andrew Taylor 39
Stokes, Gordon 235
Stone, Randolph 90, 92
Sutherland, William Garner 116
Sutton, Christine 344

T
T'ai chi ch'uan 127, 129–30
  breathing 133–4
  healer profile 132
  Traditional Chinese Medicine (TCM) 127
  what is Taoism? 131
  who can benefit? 130–3
Taoism 131, 133–4
tapping 339–43
Tesla, Nikola 223
The Journey 10, 284
  Netherlands 286
  training 286
  unblocking "dis-ease" 285
  what to expect 285–6
  who can benefit? 284–5
therapeutic sound therapy 191–2
  history 192–3
  Solfeggio tuning 193
  training 195

what to expect 195
who can benefit? 193–5
thermo-auricular therapy
228–9
ThetaHealing® 10, 288
healer profile 291
training 293
what to expect 290–2
who can benefit? 288–90
Thie, John 234
Tindall, John 226
Topping, Wayne 235
Touch for Health (TFH) 234
Traditional Chinese
Medicine (TCM) 12, 18,
80–2, 127, 135, 349
Chinese herbal medicine
80, 84
history 82
preventative medicine 83
training 83
what to expect 82–3
who can benefit? 82
Transcendental Meditation
(TM) 322, 324
Transformational Breath®
148–9
healer profile 150
training 150
what to expect 149–50
who can benefit? 149
tui na Chinese massage
80, 135
cupping 136, 137
gua sha 137, 138
herbal liniments 137
history 135
infantile tui na 138
moxibustion 137
therapeutic techniques
137
what to expect 137–8
who can benefit? 135–6

U
UK Council for
Psychotherapy 335
UK Polarity Therapy
Association 93
Usui, Mikao 59

V
Vedic astrology 78
Veltheim, John 10, 250,
252–3
vipassana meditation 325
Virtue, Doreen *Chakra
Clearing* 282

W
water crystals 201–3
Watts, Ellen 373
Weiss, Brian 11
Wheater, Tim 193
Wilkins, Arnold 174
Williams, Chris 367

Y
yoga 78–9, 281, 282, 322
polarity yoga 93
yoga nidra 318, 319
Young, Thomas 185–6

Z
Zeigler, Patrick 63
Zen meditation 324
Zhuangzi 125
Zimbaté 258
training 261
two main energy streams
258–60
what to expect 261
who can benefit? 260–1
Zimbaté Creed 260

Acknowledgements

My thanks go to Liz Dean, Chelsey Fox, Leanne Bryan, Jennifer Veall, and Giulia Hetherington for making the project happen and bringing it to fruition. I would also like to thank Emily Anderson and Alex Marr for their support and help; Will Gethin, who interviewed the wonderful Dr Emoto not long before he died, for his source material; Lyz Cooper and Faith Challoner-Wheatley, Sue Beer, Peter Kavanagh, David Hamilton, Mary Welford, Catherine Moffat, Lorraine Flaherty, Kenneth Sloan, Dr Borland, Judy Hall, Clare Gabriel, and Britt Toksvig-Jorgensen, all of whom contributed and helped me in pulling together the information for this book.

I should also acknowledge the important role of *Kindred Spirit* magazine. I have been contributing to this title for ten years and have been the editor for the past four, and during that time I have been lucky enough to experience and learn about a vast number of amazing healing therapies from all around the world, many of which are featured in this book.

Picture credits

Images 313; Francesco Ruggeri 197; fStop Images 226; Hans Casparius/Hulton Archive 330; Isa Foltin 87; John Beard/The Denver Post 109; John Howard 98; Jupiterimages 77; Kasia Wandycz/Paris Match 103, 104; Leemage 34; LightRocket 270; Mike Harrington 18; Photo Division/Radius Images 35; PhotoAlto/Antoine Arraou 126; Science Photo Library 205; Stills 9; Volanthevist 189; ZenShui/Alix Minde 314; courtesy **Hay House Publishing** photo StarShots 291; courtesy **Innersource.net** 245; courtesy **International BodyTalk Association** 252; © **International Feldenkrais Federation Archive** 100; **iStock** 22; agsandrew 374; Antonio_Diaz 225; botamochi 30; Cameron Strathdee 294; clu 310; DKsamco 82; dnberty 165; erlucho 368; FredfFroese 12; funduck 345; Heidi van der Westhuizen 300; humonia 230, 255; Klubovy 221; MarsBars 289; monkeybusinessimages 198; omgimages 246; photolyric 20; RuslanDashinsky 65; topnotch100 316; yogesh_more 192; Yuri_Arcurs 142; courtesy **thejourney.com** photo Mark Lapwood 284; courtesy masaru-emoto.net 200, 202; courtesy **Metatronic Life** 267; **National Library of Australia** (an22676564) 97; **Octopus Publishing Group** 16; Adrian Pope 340, 347; Lyanne Wylde 10; Mike Good 147; Russell Sadur 6, 25, 27, 79, 94, 140, 158, 277; Ruth Jenkinson 121, 125, 130, 323; **Palmer College of Chiropractic** Special Collections and Archives 45; courtesy **Professor Paul Gilbert** 353; **Quantum-Touch, Inc.** 273, 274; photo **Richard Grassie** 358; © **Robert Scherzinger** 112; **Science Photo Library** Antonia Reeve 118; Garion Hutchings 178; Henny Allis 148; Ian Hooton 210; RIA Novosti 152, 153; **Sergie Hajikakou** (systematic-kinesiology.co.uk) 233; **Shutterstock** Dean Bertoncelj 52; Adam Gregor 46; Aleksandar Mijatovic 336; Ammentorp Photography 157; Anneka 256; Ariwasabi 71; buttet 49; dencg 292; Dmitry Kalinovsky 80; Dragon Images 354; Elena Dijour 297; Elena Elisseeva 54; epicseurope 136; Eskemar 81; F Schmidt 23; haraldmuc 360; holbox 283; Image Point Fr 208; Irina Falkanfal 372; Ivan Roth 381; Kookai 173; Kzenon 175; lightwavemedia 43; Liudmyla Soloviova 11; LoloStock 332; Luna Vandoorne 370; Maridav 379; Martin Kubat 191; Mila Supinskaya 366; Monika Wisniewska 254; Mykola Komarovskyy 318; Naeblys 335; Neveshkin Nikolay 85; Nikki Zalewski 66; O Bellini 184; Payless Images 57; ra2studio 350; Robert Kneschke 327; Silkspin 265; taro911 Photographer 214; Tatiana Makotra 182; TonyV3112 129; Vasily Gureev 280; wavebreakmedia 60, 63, 116, 151, 228, 329; courtesy **Stanislav and Christina Grof Foundation** 160, 162; **SuperStock** Raith/Mauritius 21; **Thinkstockphotos** Jacob Wackerhausen 324; **TopFoto** The Granger Collection 269; **Wellcome Library, London** 38, 55′ **Wikipedia** Udo Schröter (CC-BY-SA-3) 24

Dedication

To all the therapists and practitioners, teachers, healers, and lightworkers
who have amazed, helped, and inspired me over the years.

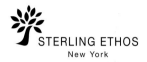

STERLING ETHOS
New York

Disclaimer

The author and publisher disclaim to any person or entity, any liability, loss, or damage
caused or alleged to be caused, directly or indirectly as a result of the use, application,
or interpretation of any of the contents of this book. All information and/or advice given
in this book should not take the place of any medical, counselling, legal, or financial
advice given to you by any qualified professional.

Claire Gillman asserts the moral right to be identified as the author of this work.

ISBN: 9781454917779

Distributed in Canada by Sterling Publishing
c/o Canadian Manda Group, 165 Dufferin Street
Toronto, Ontario, Canada M6K 3H6

For information about custom editions, special sales, and premium and corporate purchases,
please contact Sterling Special Sales at 800-805-5489 or specialsales@sterlingpublishing.com.

2 4 6 8 10 9 7 5 3 1